DATE DUE

12-9-15		
		PRINTED IN U.S.A.

ASSISTED DEATH IN EUROPE AND AMERICA

ASSISTED DEATH
IN EUROPE
AND AMERICA

Four Regimes and Their Lessons

Guenter Lewy

OXFORD
UNIVERSITY PRESS

2011

OXFORD

UNIVERSITY PRESS

Oxford University Press, Inc., publishes works that further
Oxford University's objective of excellence
in research, scholarship, and education.

Oxford   New York
Auckland   Cape Town   Dar es Salaam   Hong Kong   Karachi
Kuala Lumpur   Madrid   Melbourne   Mexico City   Nairobi
New Delhi   Shanghai   Taipei   Toronto

With offices in
Argentina   Austria   Brazil   Chile   Czech Republic   France   Greece
Guatemala   Hungary   Italy   Japan   Poland   Portugal   Singapore
South Korea Switzerland Thailand Turkey Ukraine Vietnam

Published by Oxford University Press, Inc.
198 Madison Avenue, New York, New York 10016
www.oup.com

Oxford is a registered trademark of Oxford University Press

Lewy, Guenter, 1923-
Assisted death in Europe and America : four regimes and their lessons /
by Guenter Lewy.
p. cm.
Includes bibliographical references and index.
ISBN 978-0-19-974641-5
1. Assisted suicide—Europe. 2. Assisted suicide—Oregon.
I. Title.
R726.L49 2010
179.7–dc22   2009046454

3 5 7 9 8 6 4
Printed in the United States of America
on acid-free paper

ACKNOWLEDGMENTS

The text in Appendices 1 and 2 is reprinted with permission from Paul Schotsmans and Tom Meulenbergs, eds., *Euthanasia and Palliative Care in the Low Countries* (Leuven, Belgium: Peeters, 2005).

PREFACE

At present, seven jurisdictions in the world, with various restrictions, have legalized the practice of assisted dying for those afflicted with inordinate suffering and allow physician-assisted suicide (PAS) and/or voluntary euthanasia. Three of these jurisdictions—the states of Washington and Montana in the United States, and Luxembourg in Europe—legalized assisted death during 2008 and 2009, respectively, thus providing only limited information on how these regimes will actually work. In this study I therefore concentrate on the four regimes of assisted death that have been functioning for many years and for which we have a substantial body of data, as well as observational research—the Netherlands, Belgium, and Switzerland in Europe, and Oregon in the United States. During the 1990s, PAS was legal for less than two years in the Northern Territories of Australia; four patients died under the act before the legislation was invalidated by the Australian federal parliament. I do not deal with this short-lived regime because of the limited lessons that can be derived from four cases.

Scholars write books for a variety of reasons. I undertook work on the topic of assisted death in part because I have arrived at a stage in my life when the issue of dignified and compassionate end-of-life care is of more than theoretical interest to me. Writing this book was, for me, not only a matter of addressing an issue of contemporary interest and importance but also a means of clarifying my own thinking. My attitude to assisted dying was generally sympathetic before I started work on the book, and has remained so after completion. At the same time, I have also learned of the many ways in which decisions for assisted death can go wrong, and I have become more aware of the crucial importance of adequate safeguards against abuse. That such safeguards can be instituted effectively, without being unduly onerous or undermining the discretion of doctors, is one of the important lessons gained from experience with a legalized scheme of assisted death on the part of the Netherlands, Belgium, and Oregon.

The question of how to handle end-of-life dilemmas continues to be hotly debated everywhere, and the literature on the issue is enormous. A search of PubMed for "assisted death" undertaken in 2009 yielded 7,709 citations; Google Scholar has about 760,000 references for the same subject. Most of this literature deals with the ethical, medical, or legal aspects of assisted death; a paucity of writing provides a detailed and reliable account of the way the four existing regimes are actually working, and many partisans, on both sides of the controversy, cite existing data selectively or, at times, willfully distort the empirical evidence in order to strengthen their case. Moreover, much of this literature is out-of-date because it was composed before the Netherlands and Belgium legalized voluntary euthanasia in 2002.

My purpose here is to fill this gap, and, even though I do address the lessons that can be derived from the existing regimes of assisted death in a concluding chapter, this book is largely empirical and descriptive. Facts cannot settle a moral debate. Nevertheless, accurate factual information is the precondition of any well-founded moral argument, and a largely expository and analytical study can therefore make a contribution to the philosophical debate on the issue, as well as provide guidance to the makers of public policy.

It a pleasant duty to express my gratitude for the generous assistance I have received from many quarters. A number of European scholars with expertise in the issue of assisted death took time off from their busy schedules and, in fruitful conversations and follow-up correspondence, helped me better understand the regimes their countries had instituted. In the Netherlands, I am indebted to Johannes J.M. van Delden, Agnes van der Heide, Paul J. van der Maas, M.J.P.A. Janssens, and Bregje Onwuteaka-Philipsen; in Belgium, to Lieve van den Block and Chris Gastmans; in Switzerland, to Georg Bosshard and Andreas Frei. I am grateful also to officials of organizations involved in one way or another with the issue of assisted death who made themselves available for my questions, to whit, the Association pour le droit de mourir dans la dignté in Brussels, Belgium, and the Schweizerische Gesellschaft für palliative Medizin, in Zurich, Switzerland. Special thanks are due both branches of the Swiss right-to-die organization Exit for their gracious cooperation. I had useful conversations with President Hans Wehrli-Streiff and Heidi Vogt Daeniker, head of the department *Freitodbegleitung*, of Exit— Vereinigung für humanes Sterben, Zurich. MS. Vogt also provided me with valuable documentary material. As it is customary to state, none of the above individuals or organizations are responsible for the opinions and conclusions reached in this book, which remain my personal responsibility.

Washington, D.C.
January 2010

CONTENTS

LIST OF TABLES

Tables

ABBREVIATIONS

AAHPM	American Academy of Hospice and Palliative Medicine
ALS	Amyotrophic Lateral Sclerosis (a.k.a. Lou Gehrig's disease)
ADMD	Association for the Right to Die in Dignity
BBAB	Belgian Advisory Committee on Bioethics
CAL	Commission on the Acceptability of Medical Behavior that Shortens Life
CHF	Swiss Franc
DEA	Drug Enforcement Administration
DWDA	Death with Dignity Act
EURELD	European End-of-Life Study
FPZV	Flemish Palliative Care Federation
GP	General Practitioner
KNMG	Royal Dutch Medical Association
LAWER	Life-terminating Act without Explicit Request
LEIF	Forum for End-of-Life Information
MDEL	Medical Decisions Concerning the End of Life
NaP	Natrium-Pentobarbital
NEK-CNE	National Advisory Commission on Biomedical Ethics
OSPA	Oregon State Pharmacists Association
PAS	Physician-assisted Suicide
SAMS	Swiss Academy of Medical Sciences
SAPC	Swiss Association for Palliative Care
SCEN	Support and Consultation in the Netherlands

ASSISTED DEATH IN EUROPE AND AMERICA

1

INTRODUCTION

This book deals with varieties of assisted death. Physician-assisted suicide (PAS) involves a physician helping a patient to commit suicide by providing a lethal medication. In cases of voluntary euthanasia, the physician administers or injects the lethal drug. In both types of assisted death, it is the patient—usually but not always afflicted with a terminal illness—who voluntarily seeks death, and both PAS and euthanasia therefore can be regarded as a species of suicide, most often the suicide of an inordinately suffering person near death.

Why Assisted Death Has Become an Important Public Policy Issue

The word *euthanasia,* derived from the Greek, means a "good death." Although the term euthanasia was coined in the 17th century, the idea of a "good death" has roots in classical antiquity. Many Greeks and Romans sought a painless end to their lives, and physicians often provided assistance. The Hippocratic Oath forbade the participation of physicians in acts aimed at shortening the end of life, but there is general agreement that this injunction did not represent the thinking of Greek classical society. Mainstream Greek physicians of ancient times, writes Margaret Pabst Battin, "regarded it as part of their role to provide patients whom they could not treat with a lethal drug."[1] Suicide was a widely accepted option. In the eyes of the Stoic philosophers, to live nobly also meant to die nobly, and this implied the right to choose one's moment of departure from this earth. As Seneca insisted: "The lot of man is happy, because no one continues wretched by his fault. If life pleases you, live. If not, you have a right to return whence you came."[2] Living as such is not the good, the Stoic philosopher wrote, "but living well is. The wise man therefore lives as long as he should, not as long as he can."[3]

From the fourth century on, the Christian Church strongly condemned suicide, and euthanasia was regarded as an interference with the divine prerogative to give and take life. A good death now came to be seen as that of a person who willingly and tranquilly accepted death and whatever suffering was linked to the act of dying.[4] The idea of a good Christian death—the calm acceptance of death with the moral support of family and clergy—held sway until well into the 20th century, when rapid advances in medical treatment and technology began to enable physicians to prolong life to a previously unknown extent.

Unfortunately, in many instances, these new techniques have meant not the saving of life but the prolongation of the act of dying. With the help of elaborate machinery, it is now possible to keep fatally ill patients alive in a condition that many consider worse than death. Instead of dying in one's home, surrounded by family and friends, many persons now linger for an inordinate amount of time in hospitals, sometimes practically invisible through a thicket of cables and tubes. In some cases, individuals are unconscious for weeks or even months, being kept alive by means of artificial breathing and feeding. In the eyes of many, medical technology has run out of control and often actually contributes to more suffering. Patients, it is now argued increasingly, should be entitled to choose death when pain and physical and mental deterioration undermine the possibility of a dignified and meaningful life.

An early attempt to achieve the legalization of voluntary euthanasia took place in the state of Ohio in 1906. A bill before the legislature's Committee on Medical Jurisprudence proposed that an adult of sound mind, who was suffering from extreme physical pain without hope of recovery, might petition his physician for relief. If three other physicians agreed that the case was hopeless, the patient would be put out of pain and suffering with minimum discomfort. The bill failed, and in 1937 a similar proposal died in a committee of the Nebraska legislature. A year later, in 1938, the Euthanasia Society of America was formed. The goal of the Society was to work for the legalization of euthanasia in "the belief that with adequate safeguards, the choice of immediate death rather than prolonged agony should be available to the dying."[5]

During the following years, the horrors that characterized the Nazi regime's attempt to weed out the unfit gave euthanasia a bad name. Using the "slippery slope" argument, opponents of the right to die argued that any attempt to legalize assistance in dying would inevitably lead to the elimination of the weak and disabled, as had happened in Nazi Germany. This mode of argument made no attempt to show what exactly would cause the slide to a new Nazism,[6] but the scare tactic was effective nevertheless. It was not until the 1960s that the Euthanasia Society resumed its pre-war activism. In 1967, it formed the Euthanasia Education Council that, using the slogans "Death with Dignity" and the "Right to Die," began a campaign to influence public opinion in favor of euthanasia. In an attempt to improve its image, in 1975 the Euthanasia Society of America changed its name to Society for the Right to Die, and in 1978 the Euthanasia Education Council became Concern for Dying. Two years later, Derek Humphry founded the Hemlock Society and openly advocated voluntary euthanasia and assisted suicide. The new organization grew rapidly, and by 1992 had more than 46,000 members. In 2004, the Hemlock Society changed its name to End of Life Choices, and a year later, it merged with Compassion in Dying to form what today is the largest American right-to-die organization, Compassion and Choices.

Contributing to the spread of new attitudes toward end-of-life choices has been society's emphasis on freedom of choice and the right to determine our lives to the maximum extent possible. By the late 1980s, more than 100 books and a far larger number of articles had appeared dealing with PAS and euthanasia. Courses on death and dying have proliferated on college campuses. By 1989, a survey conducted by the Chicago-based National Opinion Research Center (NORC) showed that 69% of Americans agreed with the statement that doctors should be allowed by law to end a patient's life by some painless means if the person has an incurable disease and if the patient and family request it. A year later, a Roper poll asked, "When a person has a painful and distressing terminal disease, do you think that doctors should be allowed by law to end the patient's life if there is no hope of recovery and the patient requests it?" Sixty-four percent of respondents answered this question affirmatively and only

24% were opposed. The Roper poll revealed little difference between those who identified with a religious tradition and those who did not, or among major denominations.[7]

In 1991, Humphry published his primer for suicide, *Final Exit: The Practicalities of Self-Deliverance and Assisted Suicide,* and this book remained on the *New York Times* best-seller list for 18 weeks. Within five years, *Final Exit* sold more than 600,000 copies, and there was general agreement that these sales indicated a profound shift in public attitudes toward assisted suicide. As one middle-aged woman who bought the book put it, "When I'm dying, I want to be in control."[8]

In the Cruzan case of 1990, the U.S. Supreme Court endorsed the view that the liberty protected by the due-process clause of the 14th amendment guaranteed the right of patients to refuse unwanted medical treatment, and today this and other cases have established the right of patients to hasten death by refusing to eat or drink or decline the artificial delivery of food and water.[9] This ruling has relevance for advance directives that instruct doctors on desired end-of-life care. Under the Patient Self-Determination Act of 1990, Medicare providers, such as hospitals or nursing homes, must provide patients with information about their rights under the state laws governing advance directives.[10]

Although many physicians consider advance directives such as living wills as absolutely binding, others disregard these instructions. To be sure, not all such disregard is reprehensible. There is evidence to show that preferences for various types of end-of-life treatment may vary over time. Patients often become increasingly tolerant of unpleasant states of health as their illness progresses. In view of the documented instability of the wishes expressed in advance directives, doctors may feel justified to act according to what they consider to be in the best interest of the patient.[11] Still, the fact that few physicians have been held to account for continuing aggressive treatment against the wishes of patients has added strength to the demand that patients themselves be allowed to decide when to die with dignity with the help of PAS or euthanasia.[12]

The failure of many physicians to pay adequate attention to the alleviation of pain has been another factor that has spurred interest in seeking assistance in dying. "Despite the efficacy of opioids and a commitment by the medical profession to treat pain," Timothy Quill and Diane Meier noted in an article published in 2006, "abundant evidence suggests that patients' fears of undertreatment of distressing symptoms are justified." Improvement has been made, but some physicians still worry about the danger of addiction, while others are concerned about regulatory oversight and the possibility of disciplinary action.[13] The fear of appearing after the fact to have intentionally hastened a patient's death with morphine is considered a leading cause of undertreatment of pain in terminally ill patients.[14]

Advocates of the legalization of voluntary euthanasia have used the Cruzan case to argue that the law should not stand in the way of physicians who are prepared to help patients achieve a painless and dignified death. However, so far, the courts have rejected this argument, and euthanasia remains illegal in all jurisdictions. In two decisions handed down in 1997, the Supreme Court did leave states free to enact laws allowing PAS,[15] and in October of the same year, Oregon became the first state of the union to legalize PAS. In 2008, the state of Washington followed suit and enacted a law modeled on the Oregon Death with Dignity Act. On December 5, 2008, a Montana judge ruled that, under the state constitution, a terminally ill cancer patient in Billings had a right to die with dignity and that physicians in the state can prescribe a lethal medication for self-administration by the patient.[16] On appeal, the Supreme Court of Montana, voting 4-to-3, upheld this decision on December 31, 2009, but sidestepped the broader question of whether PAS is a right guaranteed under the state constitution. Instead, the Court's narrow majority ruled that a statute passed in 1985 that addressed the withdrawal of treatment for terminally ill patients shielded a physician from prosecution for helping to hasten the death of consenting, rational, terminal patient. The Montana legislature, where passions over the issue run high, most likely will now take up the matter of PAS.[17]

In the eyes of some members of the American right-to-die movement, the fact that the existing regimes restrict PAS to terminal patients (with less than 6 months to live) leaves some badly off patients without recourse. Individuals afflicted with slowly developing degenerative neurological illnesses such as Parkinson's disease, multiple sclerosis, amyotrophic lateral sclerosis (Lou Gehrig's disease), and others may want to end their life because of intolerable suffering and loss of dignity, but unless their condition is diagnosed as terminal they do not qualify for PAS under these acts.

The fact that, until 1997, PAS was illegal in all states of the union, and the difficulties experienced especially by nonterminal patients in obtaining aid in dying, explains the phenomenon of the one-man assisted suicide practice of Dr. Jack Kevorkian, who, between 1990 and 1998, facilitated the suicide of 93 persons. The great majority of these people were not terminally ill but nevertheless were desperate for relief. There was, for example, the case of Meriam Frederick, who for four years suffered from ALS and whose terrible situation has been described by her daughter in an article published in the *New England Journal of Medicine.* Toward the end, this 72-year-old woman had lost all speech, the ability to support her head, and the ability to swallow. Three times she almost choked to death. Both mother and daughter would have preferred a death other than the one finally arranged secretly in the barren apartment of Dr. Kevorkian, but no legal help was available.[18]

Dr. Kevorkian is a pathologist with no special expertise in end-of-life care, and he generally had only a superficial knowledge of his patients' medical history. His conduct invited every conceivable abuse and probably represented the worst-case scenario of a maverick doctor acting on his own.[19] Dr. Kevorkian's willingness to help people in distress without much ado was similar to that of the anonymous gynecology resident who, in an article published in the *Journal of the American Medical Association* described how, after being woken from sleep and "bumping sleepily against walls and corners," gave a lethal injection of morphine sulfate to 20-year-old "Debbie" who was dying of ovarian cancer. The resident found the young woman suffering from severe air hunger despite nasal oxygen, vomiting unrelentingly, and asking to "get this over with."[20]

Both the cases of Dr. Kevorkian and that of "Debbie" involved unacceptable conduct, but they were also were a symptom of a medical care system gone seriously wrong in its handling of end-of-life dilemmas. In the absence of legal PAS or euthanasia, suffering patients will either manage to find an empathic and courageous physician who will help them in their hour of desperate need, or they will be tempted to resort to violent forms of suicide like jumping off the roof, blowing out their brains, or using rat poison.

Impatient with the pace of legislative change, and in order to aid non-terminal patients eager to end their life, in September 2004 a group of former Hemlock Society members founded the Final Exit Network. "With the Network's compassionate guidance and support," the president of this organization, Ted Goodwin, has stated, "physically and mentally competent adults in all 50 states are free to exercise their last human right—the right to a peaceful, dignified death."[21] Members pay an annual fee of $50. Volunteers provide counseling, training, and support; there is no charge for the support the organization provides its members. The means of death usually is helium, freely available without a doctor's prescription. When inhaled in place of oxygen, helium gas is said to result in a quick loss of consciousness and death within 15 minutes.[22]

Even though assisting suicide is illegal in most states, the courts have generally shown compassion in cases of mercy killing, and there have been few convictions for PAS. For example, when a patient of Dr. Timothy Quill committed suicide with the help of sleeping pills the doctor had provided, local prosecutors brought the case to a Rochester grand jury (assisting suicide is a felony in the state of New York), but the jurors refused to indict Quill.[23] Until recently, the work of the Final Exit Network, too, had not run into legal trouble. On February 25, 2009, however, agents of the Georgia Bureau of Investigation arrested four volunteers of the Final Exit Network and charged them with assisting the suicide of John Celmer, a member of the organization. The president of Final Exit Network has denied that the network encourages or assists suicide in any way. "Members who avail themselves of the Exit Guide Program must be capable of performing every required function without assistance of any type."[24] The outcome of this case will turn on whether the action of the organization is judged to be guidance about how to end one's life or active assistance in the act of suicide, a distinction on which there is little case law so far.[25]

Critics note that these self-help schemes do not provide for any professional evaluation of mental competency or constancy of the request for assisted death, and in fact aim at taking physicians out of the picture altogether. "The flouting of current social controls around end-of-life decisions," writes one student of what he calls the *deathing counterculture*, "is cause for serious concern."[26]

Physicians sympathetic to the suffering of seriously ill patients have responded to the absence of legal PAS and euthanasia in all but two states by making their own ad hoc life-and-death decisions. It has been estimated that 70% of the approximately 1.7 million people who die in U.S. hospitals annually die as a result of someone's decision to withhold or withdraw life-sustaining medical interventions.[27] This decision not to start or to withdraw treatment is made in full awareness of its life-shortening effect, and this fact appears to call into question the distinction made by some ethicists between killing and letting die.[28] The willingness to accept the shortening of the lives of terminal patients is even more pronounced in the various forms of sedation, a morally ambiguous set of procedures that is inadequately categorized as either ameliorative (palliative) or terminal.[29] According to the traditional Catholic principle of *double effect*, one may perform an action with a bad effect provided one foresees but does not intend the bad effect, and a secularized version of this doctrine has been invoked to allow physicians to administer heavy doses of morphine to terminally ill patients. In these situations, it is argued, the physician knows that the morphine will depress respiration and make death occur earlier, but since the doctor only seeks to relieve suffering and does not want to cause death, his action is permissible.[30] Our discussion of the Dutch experience of euthanasia will show how these dilemmas are dealt with in actual life situations.

Another way of handling hopelessly sick patients is the posting of do-not-resuscitate orders that allow patients to die without last-ditch efforts at resuscitation. The deliberate ending of life is, of course, the purpose of the PAS and euthanasia that, as we will see presently, occurs in the United States despite its clear illegality in most jurisdictions. Information available about this entirely unregulated aspect of medicine reveals a pattern that not only is secretive and deceptive, but also has great potential for abuse.

The Euthanasia and Assisted-Suicide Underground

Several studies are available of the occurrence of assisted death in the United States, all done at a time when euthanasia and PAS were illegal in all states of the union. Some of these surveys, as Ezekiel Emanuel has pointed out, are problematic in their methods. Physicians providing end-of-life care often are confused about relief that shortens life, sometimes calling it euthanasia and sometimes referring to it simply as pain relief.[31] Still, although the data on the actual frequency of euthanasia and PAS show some variation, there can be no doubt that both modes of aid in dying are practiced by physicians, as well as by nurses.

A survey of oncologists done in 1993 showed that 57.2% had received a request for euthanasia or PAS. Almost 2% had actually performed euthanasia, and 13.5% had engaged in PAS. Altogether, 13.6% of all oncologists (almost 1 in 7) had performed one of these two ways of assisted death.[32] Somewhat different rates were found in a study of Washington state physicians. Done in late 1994 and early 1995, this survey found that 26% of doctors had been asked at least once for PAS or euthanasia, and 16% had been asked more than once. These physicians had provided PAS to 24% of the patients requesting PAS and euthanasia.[33] Last, a 1996 national survey of specialists likely to deal with dying patients showed that 3.3% of these physicians had written at least one prescription for PAS, and 4.7% had administered at least one lethal injection.[34]

Nurses, too, have been found to be involved with both PAS and euthanasia. A study of oncology nurses published in 1997 showed that 30% had received a request for assistance in dying and 25% a request for euthanasia. One percent of these nurses had actually participated in assisted suicide, and 4.5% had performed euthanasia.[35] Summing it all up, Timothy Quill and his co-authors write: "Studies in the United States consistently show the existence of an underground, illegal practice that is undocumented and unregulated, lacks the benefit of a second opinion, is not prosecuted, and is not rare."[36] Quill stresses that this covert practice of assisted death is "dangerous for patients and erodes the integrity of the professions of medicine and law."[37]

Australian doctor Roger S. Magnusson has studied the euthanasia underground that has developed especially in the care of patients with human immunodeficiency virus/acquired immune deficiency syndrome (HIV/AIDS). Using interviews with health care professionals in Sidney, Melbourne, and San Francisco, Magnusson found an environment of secrecy characterized by frequent "botched attempts" to perform euthanasia; evidence of coercion upon the patient, and/or the health care worker; evidence of rash or hasty involvement by doctors with little or no knowledge of the patient's circumstances; evidence of euthanasia upon able-bodied patients who are not in the terminal stages of illness; and an all-pervasive culture of deception.

Magnusson's indictment, based on these findings, is harsh:

> The surreptitious practice of euthanasia illustrates, in many ways, the very opposite of those attributes which characterize "medical professionalism." In the euthanasia underground there is no specialized training. Participants remain ignorant about what is needed to achieve a gentle death. There is a proliferation of what participants refer to bluntly as "botched attempts." Accountability is also absent. The medical profession for the most part turns a blind eye to the practice of illicit euthanasia by its members. There are no norms or principles guiding involvement. Rather, participation is shrouded in secrecy and deception, triggered by highly idiosyncratic factors, with evidence of casual and precipitative involvements. In place of a tradition of disinterested service to patients, there is evidence of a complete lack of "professional distance," sharp conflicts of interest, and examples of euthanasia without consent.[38]

Magnusson reported frequent botched attempts to perform euthanasia, and we have other, anecdotal, accounts of assisted suicide gone awry. Patients either vomited the medication or the doses where insufficient, so that family members or others eventually had to end the patient's life by asphyxiation with a pillow or a plastic bag.[39] As we will see in subsequent chapters, such unfortunate events are far less likely to occur when PAS is performed by physicians trained in the proper methods of bringing about a quick and complication-free death.

The disturbing thing about this euthanasia underground, Magnusson added, was that, for the most part, it did not involve a freakish fringe but the practice of respected and experienced professionals. Moreover, although the Australian researcher's study was focused on the fate of AIDS patients, Magnusson thought it unlikely that this underground, with all of its many abuses, was limited to one class of patients.[40] This conclusion is supported by data from other studies. In his survey of critical care nurses, David Asch calculated that at least 7% of the nurses interviewed had at least once carried out assisted suicide or euthanasia without a request from either the patient or a surrogate. Another 4% had hastened a patient's death by only pretending to provide the life-sustaining treatment ordered by a physician. Some nurses reported engaging in these practices without a request or advance knowledge of physicians.[41]

Similar failures of professionalism are reported for physicians. In his study of Washington doctors' responses to requests for PAS or euthanasia, Back found that patients received a second opinion, a generally accepted essential safeguard, in only 15% of the cases.[42] The national survey of physicians conducted by Meier and her co-authors revealed that 54% of the patients who received a lethal injection did not make the request for euthanasia themselves. The majority of these patients, the researchers reported, had less than 24 hours to live. However, even under these circumstances, the rate of involuntary cases of euthanasia appears to be high.[43]

Another major problem arises from the well-documented frequent failure of physicians to diagnose the presence of depression. Surveying the literature on this subject, Nico Peruzzi and his co-authors have concluded: "The capacity of physicians untrained in psychiatry to diagnose depression is alarmingly low (varying from 20% to 60% in these studies)."[44] Depression is a condition known to be a contributing factor in the desire for hastened death, while at the same time it often also leads to impaired competence in making requests for aid in dying. As we will see in the following chapters, even legally controlled programs of PAS and euthanasia so far have done poorly in dealing with this issue. It is an especially serious problem in the completely unregulated underground practice of PAS and euthanasia, where patients rarely have the benefit of even a physician's second opinion.

Many seriously ill patients express hopelessness about their condition, but not every hopeless patient is clinically depressed. Terminal patients may be profoundly sad, and even feel depressed, due to a realistic appraisal of their condition, and this may create a heightened desire to hasten death. The distinction between such a pessimistic outlook, which, on the one hand, may lead a patient to devalue the possible benefits of life-extending treatment, and, on the other hand, a treatable clinical depression, is difficult to make, especially for physicians without psychiatric training. An additional difficulty is the fact, noted by one expert, "that both patients and physicians may also be reluctant to invite the additional scrutiny, and intrusion, that a label of depression might entail, leading both parties to avoid discussing, acknowledging, or addressing possible depressive symptoms."[45] Moreover, even in cases in which depression is found to be present, it is not known how severe the depression must be before it precludes rational judgment and justifies the diagnosis of incompetence.[46]

The difficulties in the diagnosis of depression and the complex nature of this disorder have led to the suggestion that all patients desiring assistance in dying be required to undergo a psychiatric evaluation and pass a "psychiatric filter."[47] But even those who do not insist on a compulsory psychiatric examination—because of its potentially humiliating impact or because they do not want psychiatrists to be gatekeepers for patients seeking assisted death—stress the crucial importance of a waiting period and some screening measures for depression.[48] A 2001 study of nonterminal patients seeking PAS or euthanasia showed that between 8% and 26% of such patients reversed their preference after 6 months—most often in the direction of late rejection. Even depressed patients in despair have been known to reverse their wish for death. The authors of this study therefore stressed the importance of a mental health evaluation and a waiting period to ensure that the desire for death is persistent.[49] Such procedures can be implemented in regimes that impose careful procedural controls on PAS and euthanasia. They very obviously cannot be realized in an illegal and completely unregulated underground environment.

Neil Gorsuch is correct in pointing out that evidence about the pervasiveness of the clandestine practice of PAS and euthanasia "can be wielded by partisans on both sides of the debate—constituting to some a reason for greater vigilance and enforcement rather than a reason for legalization."[50] On strictly theoretical grounds, it can indeed be argued that better laws and better enforcement of existing laws might end or at least decrease the frequency of various illegal forms of assisted death. And yet, actual experience over many years in both the United States and Europe casts doubt on this expectation. Margaret Otlowski has looked into the effectiveness of legal controls in various countries, and has concluded that criminal prohibitions fail to control euthanasia. The question, therefore, is probably not whether to permit PAS and euthanasia. The real "choice we face is whether we seek to regulate and control the practice of euthanasia or whether it is left unregulated and unchecked, which creates greater risks for both doctors and patients."[51]

The Aims of This Study

Support for PAS and euthanasia has increased steadily in the United States (and in Europe). "Studies conducted over the past decade," noted Barry Rosenfeld in 2000, "have consistently demonstrated a substantial majority approval (roughly two thirds of respondents) of legalization for some form of assisted suicide or euthanasia."[52] This trend has continued, as can be seen in the approval of PAS in Washington state in 2008. Similar ballot initiatives are under way in California, Michigan, and Maine. Public opinion alone, as measured in surveys, probably should not decide the question of the legalization of assisted death, but this is not to deny the validity of referenda that have led to the legalization of PAS in Oregon and Washington. These actions took place after a lengthy campaign that highlighted the various social and moral complexities that must be addressed. Without such a program of public education, voters cannot be expected to make an intelligent and responsible choice.

In this book, I do not intend to undertake an in-depth analysis of the substantive arguments that support or oppose assisted death, the subject of a vast literature that hardly needs further enlargement. As stated in the preface, the approach of this work is descriptive and empirical. Knowledge gained in such an endeavor can play a constructive role in the continuing dialogue on assisted death.

The discussion of moral issues is often conducted on the basis of fundamental values and ethical principles, such as justice, right action, moral duty, or moral obligation (what philosophers call *deontological arguments*). With regard to PAS and euthanasia, the most common such argument, that of opposing all forms of assisted death, affirms the intrinsic value of human life and maintains that no private person is ever allowed to end it. Thus, for example, the "Declaration on Euthanasia," issued by the Vatican's Sacred Congregation for the Doctrine of the Faith on May 5, 1980, states that life is a gift of God and that suicide is, therefore, as wrong as murder. Suffering is held to have a "special place in God's saving plan," although the principle of the double effect allows the alleviation of pain and suffering, even at the risk of shortening life.[53] Neil Gorsuch similarly maintains that human life is "fundamentally and inherently valuable" and that therefore "the intentional taking of human life by private persons is always wrong."[54] This position is further strengthened by the argument that it is the physician's duty to "do no harm" and that this duty therefore forbids the doctor's participation in any form of PAS or euthanasia. The most important deontological argument in favor of PAS and euthanasia is based on the principle of respect for autonomy. Suffering patients are held to have the right to determine and control the time, place, and nature of their death, and PAS and voluntary euthanasia are therefore seen as a basic human right.[55]

In the nature of the case, deontological arguments are extremely difficult to resolve or reconcile, especially when they are based on theological premises but also when they invoke basis human rights. A discussion of PAS and euthanasia based exclusively on this mode of moral argument is unlikely to lead to the kind of compromise that often is necessary in the development of public policy. On the other hand, consequentialist arguments that invoke the consequences of a given course of action, I believe, will more easily provide a basis for policy, a policy that can be supported by men and women of good will who do not necessarily agree on fundamental beliefs such as whether human life is a gift of God or whether it is ever right to kill.

Gorsuch is correct in insisting that consequentialist arguments in and by themselves cannot solve moral issues and predicaments: "Endeavoring to compare or weigh, say, the interest the rational adult tired with life has in choosing death against the interest the incompetent elderly widow has in avoiding being killed by a greedy guardian and heir, without reference to any extrinsic agreed-upon moral rule or code is a seemingly impossible, even senseless, enterprise." It is senseless in the same way as it is senseless to compare the virtues of apples and oranges.[56] And yet, it is the great advantage of consequentialist arguments that, unlike deontological ones, they can be analyzed empirically.

Empirical evidence can be collected about the frequency with which rational adults afflicted with an insufferable illness will seek assistance in dying and how often it happens that incompetent women are put to death at the urging of greedy next-of-kin. Given the extensive experience with legal forms of PAS and euthanasia in several countries, is there evidence to indicate that these societies are sliding down the "slippery slope" toward a general loss of respect for human life? Evidence can be adduced for or against the validity of assertions, such as that the availability of PAS or euthanasia reduces the anxiety of patients fearful of a prolonged and agonizing process of dying or that it leads to a disproportionate number of assisted suicides among the uneducated and poor. Given an agreement that the avoidance of inordinate suffering is good and desirable and that the abuse of incompetent persons is bad and should be avoided—and such an agreement can surely be assumed—it then becomes possible to develop a public policy that will promote these agreed-upon ends, and one that includes safeguards against abuse.

I do not wish to minimize the difficulty of such an undertaking. As a task force on PAS of the Society for Health and Human Values correctly noted in an important report published in 1995, the adequacy of safeguards may be challenged as being either too permissive and therefore leading to a "slippery slope" problem, or as so restrictive that they entangle suffering patients in lengthy bureaucratic procedures. Is it possible to devise safeguards and procedures that are sufficiently flexible to respond to the individual circumstances of the patient and the illness, and yet sufficiently strict so as to protect vulnerable populations? "Assuming that no human system can be error-free, how great an error rate is acceptable in such a system of policing?"[57]

There is also the well-known complexity of any cost–benefit analysis. Much depends upon the validity of the instruments with which relevant data are collected and on the quality of the analysis of these data. And yet, as the Dutch scholar Johannes M. van Delden has correctly stressed, while "facts will not settle a moral debate," one cannot do ethics properly unless one knows the facts correctly.[58] It is in line with this principle that my aim in this book is to provide a reliable fact-based analysis of the way that PAS and euthanasia actually operates in several different societies and to suggest what can be learned from this knowledge.

2

EUTHANASIA AND PHYSICIAN-ASSISTED SUICIDE IN THE NETHERLANDS

Until 2002, Article 293 of the Dutch criminal code prohibited the killing of a person at his or her request, and Article 294 forbade assisting someone to commit suicide. Yet despite these unequivocal legal provisions criminalizing all forms of assisted death, a series of court cases over time had made both voluntary euthanasia and physician-assisted suicide (PAS) a practice that carried little risk of prosecution. Legalization, when it came in 2002, for the most part merely changed the law to make it conform to what had long become accepted by the public, the medical profession, and the courts.

The Path to Legalization

Advances in medical care in the developed world have greatly extended the life span but have also often meant a lengthy dying process, unduly prolonged with the help of various technical gadgets. Many physicians have adjusted to this new situation by quietly ending life-prolonging treatments for patients with no chance of recovery, or at times even disconnecting life-sustaining machinery, and this includes physicians in the Netherlands. However, the Dutch people's inherent pragmatism, search for consensus, and willingness to confront difficult situations frankly has led also to the use of more active measures to assist the dying of ill patients who are suffering unbearably.[1]

Several developments in Dutch society help explain the gradual acceptance of assisted death, and among these is the family-oriented Dutch health care system. Dutch general practitioners generally serve an entire family, taking care of the family's health care needs over the course of a lifetime, and acting as attending physicians in family members' deaths. Because they are closely involved with their patients over a long period of time—including during the dying process—Dutch doctors have increased willingness to help their charges achieve a less stressful and more comfortable death.

As in the rest of the Western world, the 1960s in the Netherlands were a time of increased preoccupation with personal autonomy and self-assertion. The churches saw a diminishing of their influence, and people claimed a greater role in all decisions affecting life and death. This, then, was the background for the public debate that began in the early 1970s and centered on the role of the physician in difficult end-of-life situations. In 1969, psychiatrist/neurologist Dr. J.H. van den Berg published a book arguing for the adjustment of medical ethics to the new medical realities. Van den Berg maintained that, although it was the duty of doctors to preserve and extend life, sometimes the prolongation of life made no sense.[2] Van den Berg's book was widely discussed in the media and was reprinted 21 times within seven years. Obviously it had confronted a topic of major importance to the Dutch public.

During these years, several organizations and political parties came out in favor of allowing doctors, in exceptional cases, to help hopelessly ill and greatly suffering patients to end their life. This was the recommendation of the Dutch Humanist Society and of the right-of-center People's Party for Freedom and Democracy. In 1975, a working group of the Royal Dutch Medical Association (KNMG), the professional association of Dutch doctors, issued a report that accepted active euthanasia in those rare cases in which no other relief from great suffering was possible. In 1978, the Committee on Legislation of the Dutch Association for Voluntary Euthanasia, founded in 1973, proposed a change in Article 293 of the criminal code that would allow active euthanasia by a doctor when three conditions had been met: a fully informed patient had made a voluntary, well-considered and unequivocal request for euthanasia; the patient was in a terminal condition; and the euthanasia was performed by the doctor responsible for the patient's treatment.[3]

The emerging consensus was also reflected in a number of court decisions. In 1971, Dr. Geertruda Postma had ended the life of her 78-year-old mother, who was deaf, partly paralyzed, bound to a wheelchair in a nursing home, and had repeatedly pleaded for release from her suffering. Dr. Postma injected her mother with a fatal dose of morphine, and in February 1973, she was tried in the district court of Leeuwarden for "killing on request," a violation of Article 293 of the criminal code. The medical inspector testified that, under certain conditions, doctors no longer considered it necessary to prolong a patient's life endlessly, and the court, while finding Dr. Postma guilty under the law, appeared to agree with this view. It handed down a suspended sentence of one week's imprisonment and one year's probation.[4]

Eight years later, there followed an even more important decision by the district court in Rotterdam, in the *Wertheim* case in November 1981. A voluntary euthanasia activist had helped a 67-year-old woman, who suffered from many ailments of both a physical and mental nature, to commit suicide. The court ruled that assistance with suicide could be justified in certain special circumstances:

- The suffering of the person was unbearable.
- Both the suffering and the desire to die were enduring.
- The decision to die was voluntary.
- The person was aware of and had considered available alternatives.
- No alternatives to improve the situation were available.
- The person's death did not cause unnecessary suffering to others.

The assistance to die itself, the court decided, had to meet the following requirements:

- More than one person had to be involved in the decision.
- The assistance had to be provided by a physician.
- The decision had to be made with the utmost care, which included a consultation with another doctor and with a specialist if the patient's condition was not yet terminal.

Because Ms. Wertheim was not a physician and therefore had not met these requirements, she was found guilty of the offense of assisting suicide. Following this case, the college of procurators-general, the body that sets public policy for all public prosecutions, decided that all cases involving Article 293 (euthanasia) and Article 294 (assisted suicide) were to be referred to the college for a decision on whether to prosecute. The aim was to achieve uniformity based on the guidelines contained in the *Postma* and *Wertheim* cases.[5]

The *Schoonheim* case, which began in the district court of Alkmaar in 1983, further clarified the legal situation regarding euthanasia and assisted suicide. Dr. Schoonheim, a general practitioner, had performed euthanasia on a frail 95-year-old woman who was bedridden due to a fractured hip, had dizzy spells, had lost much of her ability to see and hear, suffered greatly from her condition of dependency, and repeatedly had requested her doctor to end her life. The district court accepted the argument of Schoonheim's lawyer that his client had acted in a situation of *overmacht* (justification due to necessity or *force majeure*), and this claim was eventually upheld by the Supreme Court. Article 40 of the Dutch criminal code provides that a person is not guilty of a criminal offense if the action was "the result of a force he could not be expected to resist [*overmacht*]." This provision has been interpreted to apply to situations of necessity in which an actor made a justifiable choice between two conflicting duties. In this case, the Supreme Court held, the physician on one hand had the duty to respect life (as laid down in Articles 293 and 294), but on the other hand, he also had the duty to relieve suffering or respect a patient's autonomy. Hence, a physician who, in line with prevailing norms of medical ethics, opted for the latter course had acted in a manner that was justifiable and had not committed a criminal act.[6] This legal principle remained in force until the legalization of euthanasia in 2002.

While the Supreme Court deliberated on the *Schoonheim* case in 1984, the executive board of the KNMG, joined by the Association of Nurses and Nurses Aides, in August of that year adopted a new policy statement on euthanasia, defined as "conduct that is intended to terminate another person's life at his or her explicit request." Given this definition, the policy statement covered both euthanasia as well as assisted suicide. According to the statement, euthanasia performed by a physician should be considered acceptable when the doctor had taken steps to meet five "requirements of careful practice":

1. The patient's request for euthanasia is voluntary and not the result of pressure from others. A written declaration will help establish voluntariness.

2. The request is well-considered, based on an awareness of alternative solutions, and repeated at least once.
3. The patient's desire for death is persistent and not the result of a temporary depression.
4. The patient experiences his suffering as persistent, unbearable, and hopeless, and is unable to die in a dignified manner. The physician should verify that these criteria are met through intensive and repeated conversations with the patient.
5. The physician has to consult at least one colleague about the request of the patient.

The statement noted that, although nurses and nursing aides often are closely involved in euthanasia activities, both the decision for and the execution of euthanasia must be in the hands of a physician. Given the possibility of unforeseen complications during the dying process, the physician should be available during the entire procedure. A doctor who is morally opposed to euthanasia should refer the patient to another provider.[7]

A year later, in August 1985, the State Commission on Euthanasia, created by Queen Beatrix in 1982, issued a report that broadly followed the recommendations of both the courts and the KNMG in laying out the conditions under which voluntary euthanasia would be permissible. The Commission proposed a revision of Article 293 to make euthanasia legal when performed by a doctor at the request of a hopelessly ill patient "in the context of careful medical practice." For the cases of persons who cannot make their wishes known, the Commission proposed a new article (292b), which allowed euthanasia for patients in irreversible coma and whose medical treatment had been stopped because it was futile. Two members filed a minority report in which they rejected any legalization of euthanasia.[8] Also that year, the KNMG appointed a Commission on the Acceptability of Medical Behavior That Shortens Life, which eventually delivered four reports dealing with patients unable or not competent to request euthanasia, minors, defective newborns, and persons suffering from mental illness. I will return to these subjects later in this chapter.

The *Admiraal* case, decided in 1985, finally made it clear that a doctor who complied with the requirements of "careful medical practice" would not be found guilty and convicted for performing euthanasia. In November 1983, the anesthetist Admiraal had ended the life of a patient suffering from multiple sclerosis who suffered greatly from her complete loss of independence and repeatedly had requested to die. Even though Admiraal had failed to consult an expert on multiple sclerosis, the court concluded that he had carefully weighed his conflicting duties, had made a justifiable choice, and had complied with the requirements of careful practice. The precedent-setting nature of this decision was confirmed by the Minister of Justice, who informed the Medical Association in September 1985 that a doctor who fulfilled the "requirements of careful practice" would not be prosecuted for euthanasia.[9]

Some legislators felt that the issue of euthanasia should not be left to prosecutors and judges, and that parliament should end the legal insecurity of both doctors and patients by passing an appropriate law revising Articles 293 and 294 of the criminal code. In 1986, the government referred the matter to the Council of State, a crown-appointed body that must be consulted before the cabinet submits legislation to the parliament. The Council of State advised that, in its view, the public discussion on euthanasia had not yet reached the point that justified the legalization of euthanasia. After soliciting additional views from the Health Council (an independent group charged with providing advice on matters of public health) and the Assembly (or Board) of Procurators-General (a body operating under the direction of the Minister of Justice that sets policy for all public prosecutors), at the end of 1987 the government proposed amending the Law on Medical Practice to incorporate the criteria for careful medical practice in cases of euthanasia but to leave the criminal code unchanged.[10]

There followed in short order several further incremental adjustments. In November 1990, the Procurators-General issued new instructions concerning the police investigation of reported cases of euthanasia. There had been complaints about policemen arriving with sirens screaming and bursting into hospital wards or offices, and about the long interrogations to which doctors and the family of the deceased were subjected. The police now were advised to be as discrete as possible. When visiting a doctor in the course of an investigation, they were not to be in uniform, and they were to respect the feelings of next of kin.[11]

Also in 1990, the Ministry of Justice and the executive board of the KNMG agreed upon a new reporting procedure for cases of euthanasia that aimed at harmonizing differing regional prosecution policies. Physicians were to report instances of euthanasia to the local medical examiner by means of a lengthy questionnaire. The medical examiner then reported these cases to the local district attorney (prosecutor), but as long as the physician had complied with the requirements of careful medical practice, he would not be prosecuted.[12]

After the so-called Remmelink Report of 1991 had provided detailed information on the way euthanasia and assisted suicide were actually working, the government proposed and, in December 1993, parliament approved an amendment to the Law on the Disposal of Corpses (also known as the Burial Act) that went into effect in 1994. It created a new form for the reporting of cases of euthanasia that included a list of "points requiring attention" and that were to be covered in the doctor's report to the coroner (medical examiner). These points largely corresponded to the requirements of careful practice affirmed in earlier court decisions.[13]

The 1994 law provided formal legal status to the reporting procedures that had been in use since 1991. To ensure uniformity of treatment, the coroner was to report cases of euthanasia to the public prosecutor of the district in which they took place. The latter then presented his assessment to the prosecutor general (the head of a multidistrict area), who in turn reported to the five-member Assembly of Procurators-General. This body made a preliminary decision whether to prosecute, then referred the case to the minister of justice for final action. Although not legalizing euthanasia, parliament in effect thus ratified the legal principles and procedures governing allowable euthanasia that the courts had approved and which various agreements had prescribed over many years.[14]

A study published in 1997 showed that the number of cases referred to the Assembly of Prosecutors-General was small—120 out of a total of 6,324 cases during the years 1991–1995 (about 0.2%)—and that the number of cases actually prosecuted was smaller still—a total of 13 physicians during the same period. The absence of an explicit request from the patient appeared to be have been the most important reasons for these punitive proceedings.[15]

In another attempt to decrease the role of criminal law in cases of euthanasia, in January 1997, the government proposed an amendment to the 1994 law. It established five regional multidisciplinary review committees to review each case of euthanasia reported to the medical examiner. The committees were to be composed of a lawyer, a physician, and an ethicist, and were given the function of advising the public prosecutor on the question of whether to charge or dismiss a reported case. It was expected that the existence of these committees would increase the willingness of physicians to report cases of euthanasia, a matter of serious concern to which I will return. The government also proposed two different notification procedures—one for cases of voluntary euthanasia and another for cases in which the patient's life had been ended without the patient's explicit consent. The Dutch parliament approved these changes in the fall of 1997, and they became effective in 1998.[16]

One of the requirements of "careful practice" in regard to euthanasia has always been the need to consult a second physician, and most doctors report that they do so. A survey of family doctors published in 1992 showed that three-quarters of general practitioners (GPs) did seek a second opinion; in 28% of these cases, the physician consulted was a specialist.[17] In an attempt to improve the quality of this consultation, in 1997, the KNMG established the Support and Consultation on Euthanasia in Amsterdam (SCEA) project. Under this program, GPs received special training in giving advice to colleagues in matters involving euthanasia. After a positive evaluation in 1999, it was decided to set up a nationwide network of consultants, and the name of the project was changed to Support and Consultation in the Netherlands (SCEN). A study published in 2004 showed that, by the end of 2002, a total of 495 physicians had successfully completed the training program, and there were six SCEN physicians per 100 GPs. Between April 2000 and December 2002, SCEN physicians were contacted 3,891 times for a formal consultation to assess whether the requirements of "careful practice" had been met, and 643 times for informal information and advice.[18]

The SCEN program is said to have enhanced the significance of the consultation required before euthanasia can take place. A 1992 study had shown that family doctors usually consulted a partner in their practice, and only in 5% of the cases did they seek a second opinion from a doctor they did not know personally.[19] On the other hand, when a GP contacts the SCEN program, he does not know who the on-duty SCEN physician will be, and this guarantees the independence of the consultant, who usually turns out to be more stringent in his assessment. SCEN physicians gave a negative judgment in 30% of the requests even though, according to the attending doctor, all criteria for careful practice had been met. Other consultants issued a negative opinion only in 9% of the cases presented to them.

Eighty-five percent of physicians who had performed euthanasia during the period studied had contacted SCEN for consultation and/or information and advice, and practically all reported to have benefited from doing so. General practitioners singled out the expertise and accessibility of the consultant as particularly helpful. The criteria of due care necessarily are phrased in general terms, which produces some vagueness. A consultant with extensive experience will find it easier to apply general principles to concrete cases and thus will be able reduce the legal insecurity experienced by doctors when making their decision. The SCEN program is now being expanded to hospitals and nursing homes.[20]

The Law of 2002 Decriminalizing Euthanasia and Physician-assisted Suicide

By the end of the 1990s, voluntary euthanasia and PAS in the Netherlands had achieved the status of de facto legality; however, physicians helping their suffering patients to die were still presumed guilty until proven innocent. Large numbers of physicians still hesitated to report cases of euthanasia, and sentiment to end this anomalous situation increased. In early 1996, the Dutch Association for Voluntary Euthanasia drafted a bill that removed many of the regulatory guidelines for prudent practice that had evolved over the years. This clearly went too far, but when a more moderate private members' bill providing for legalization attracted a parliamentary majority,[21] the government decided to take the initiative and introduced legislation that eventually became law. That bill abolished criminal liability for voluntary euthanasia and PAS, and introduced several new provisions, but for the most part merely codified existing practice.

After considerable debate, the government bill was approved by the lower house of the Dutch parliament on November 28, 2000, by a vote of 104 to 40; the upper chamber followed suit on April 10, 2001, confirming the legislation by a vote of 46 to 28. The chief criticism of the new law came from the Catholic Church and several small Christian parties, but their political influence proved to be weak. In conformity with Dutch constitutional practice, the bill legalizing voluntary euthanasia and PAS was made law by a royal decree of Queen Beatrice and became effective as of April 1, 2002.[22]

The preamble of the Termination of Life on Request and Assisted Suicide (Review Procedures) Act explains the purpose of the law as the desire "to include a ground for exemption from criminal liability for the physician who, with due observance of the requirements of due care to be laid down by law, terminates a life on request or assists in the suicide of another person, and to provide a statutory notification and review procedure." The "requirements of due care" (in the literature often also called "careful practice" or "prudent care") are listed in Article 2. The law expects that the physician

a. holds the conviction that the request by the patient was voluntary and well-considered,
b. holds the conviction that the patient's suffering was lasting and unbearable,
c. has informed the patient about the situation he was in and about his prospects,
d. and the patient hold[s] the conviction that there was no other reasonable solution for the situation he was in,
e. has consulted at least one other, independent physician who has seen the patient and has given his written opinion on the requirements of due care, referred to in parts a–d, and
f. has terminated the life or assisted in a suicide with due care.

Articles 3–19 lay down the composition and duties of the five regional review committees who previously had a purely advisory role, and who now are given enhanced powers. Under the new law, these committees now function as a buffer between the physician and criminal law, a change designed to increase the willingness of doctors to report cases of euthanasia and PAS. Each committee consists of "an uneven number of members, including at any rate one legal specialist, also chairman, one physician and one expert on ethical or philosophical issues," as well as deputy members of each of these three categories (Article 3). The members of the committees are appointed by the government for a period of six years; they may be reappointed for a second final term of six years, and they may be dismissed "for reasons of unsuitability or incompetence or for other important reasons" (Articles 4–6). The committee has the task of assessing "whether the physician who has terminated a life on request or assisted in a suicide has acted in accordance with the requirements of due care, referred to in Article 2." The committee makes this decision on the basis of reports filed by the municipal coroner and the physician involved in the act of assisted death.[23] In carrying out this assignment, "where this is necessary for a proper assessment of the physician's actions," the committee "may request the physician to supplement his report in writing or verbally," and they may make inquiries of the municipal coroner, the consultant, or the providers of care (Article 8).

Within six weeks (or maximum 12 weeks) of receiving the physician's report, the committee is to inform him or her of its decision. If the physician is found to have acted in conformity with the requirements of due care, the case is closed and no further action is taken. In these cases, the termination of a person's life at his or her request (euthanasia) or PAS is treated in the same way as cases involving the cessation of or withholding of treatment that serves no medical purpose. All of these actions are considered normal medical practices that do not fall within the scope of the criminal law. Only in cases in which the physician has failed to act with due care does the committee forward the case to the Board of Procurators General, the regional health care inspector, and the public prosecutor, who will open a criminal investigation (Articles 9–10).

To enhance transparency and accountability, the committees are required to issue a joint annual report on their activities. This report must include the numbers of cases of euthanasia and assisted suicide, the nature of these cases, and the opinions and considerations involved in the decisions (Article 17).

The final provisions of the 2002 law amended existing legislation. Article 293 of the Criminal Code, which had made it illegal to terminate the life of another person at that person's request, was changed so that this action "shall not be punishable if it has been committed by a physician who has met the requirements of due care as referred to in Article 2" of the new law and who, instead of filing a certificate of death as a result of natural causes, informs the municipal medical examiner that death was the result of his assistance. The same change is made in Article 294, which had forbidden any assistance in the suicide of another or procuring the means to commit suicide (Article 20).

The Dutch Termination of Life on Request and Assisted Suicide (Review Procedures) Act of 2002, in addition to formally abolishing criminal liability for assisted death when a physician has exercised due care, also created several new provisions that expanded the practice of euthanasia. Article 2.2, allows a physician to euthanize an incompetent patient, one "no longer capable of expressing his will," if that patient has left a written advance directive requesting euthanasia in the case of unbearable suffering caused by Alzheimer's disease or similar afflictions. The physician had the duty to satisfy himself that the patient, "prior to reaching this condition was deemed to have [had] a reasonable understanding of his interests." Moreover, the existence of an advance directive does not relieve the physician from the need to comply with all the requirements of due care, such as concluding that the patient's suffering was indeed lasting and unbearable. This is in line with the basic principle underlying the legislation that patients have no absolute right to assisted death, and doctors have no absolute duty to perform it.

Article 2.3–4, allows a minor patient (younger than 18 years) to request assistance in death. For a minor who is between the ages of 16 and 18, and "who may be deemed to have a reasonable understanding of his interests," the physician may terminate the patient's life "after the parent or the parents exercising parental authority and/or his guardian have been involved in the decision process" (i.e., they must be consulted). For a minor who is between the ages of 12 and 16 and who likewise "may be deemed to have a reasonable understanding of his interests, the physician may carry out the patient's request," provided that those who exercise parental authority "agree with the termination of life or the assisted suicide."

On the other hand, the new law also tightens the requirements of due care. For example, before carrying out the act of assisted death, the physician must consult an "independent" physician; that is, a doctor who is neither connected with him nor involved in the treatment of the patient, and this consultant must see the patient and give his assessment in writing (Article 2.e).

Empirical Data on Euthanasia and Physician-assisted Suicide: Who, When, Why, Where, and How?

The Dutch government has sponsored a number of studies that provide demographic and other data on the practice of what are called medical decisions concerning the end of life (MDEL). In addition to data on euthanasia and PAS, these studies have included surveys on nontreatment (withholding or withdrawal of treatment) and the administration of high dosages of opioids, even if these have the effect of hastening death. The first of these nationwide investigations was commissioned in 1990, and carried out by Professor Paul van der Maas of Erasmus University of Rotterdam. Made public in September 1991, the study was called the Remmelink Report, named after Professor J. Remmelink, the attorney general of the Dutch Supreme Court, who chaired the commission to which the report was presented.[24] Broadly similar studies have since been repeated in 1995, 2001, and 2005.[25] An official evaluation of the 2002 law legalizing euthanasia and PAS was published in May 2007,[26] and several other less-comprehensive studies have been carried out dealing with various aspects of the practice of euthanasia and PAS.

One of the important aims of these investigations has been to arrive at a reliable estimate of the actual incidence of euthanasia and PAS, since the number of officially reported cases was known to be incomplete. The methodology employed to find this information has included:

- Interviews with a stratified sample of 405 physicians from different disciplines, including GPs, nursing-home doctors, and physicians in specialities such as cardiology and internal medicine, who together attend the great majority of deaths in the Netherlands. (The 2005 study did not make use of these interviews.)
- A study of 7,000 death certificates in which the cause of death included an MDEL; physicians involved in these MDELs were sent a questionnaire, under a procedure that guaranteed anonymity, in

which they were asked to answer questions about the way in which they had handled these MDELs—whether there had been a request for assisted death, whether patients had been competent to make decisions, etc. Interviews and questionnaires yielded similar results.

- A prospective study in which physicians interviewed in study 1 were asked to complete a questionnaire identical to that used in study 2 and in which they described all the deaths and the decisions they had made (or not made) during the six months after the interview. (This prospective study was used only in 1991.)
- Interviews with a sample of coroners and a study of judicial files (used in 1995).

The Minister of Justice guaranteed legal immunity in respect to all information collected in these studies, and cooperation on the part of the physicians contacted satisfied relevant standards of statistical reliability.[27]

Nontreatment decisions and the administration of opioids even though they may hasten death are commonly resorted to by physicians throughout the Western world, and I will return to the use of these practices in the Netherlands later in this chapter. For now, I focus on the figures (best estimates) of euthanasia and PAS, and these show an increase between 1990 and 1995, a leveling off in 2001, and a decrease in 2005 and 2006. The total number of requests for euthanasia and PAS rose from 8,900 in 1990 to 9,700 in 1995, held steady at 9,700 in 2001, and fell to 8,400 in 2005. Although in 2001 there were 3,500 reported cases of euthanasia and 300 cases of PAS, the corresponding numbers for 2006 had decreased to 1,765 and 132 respectively (26 cases combined the two procedures of assisted death).[28]

Since the total number of deaths in the Netherlands was not static during these years, the rate of euthanasia and PAS in relation to all deaths (Table 2.1) probably gives the most meaningful picture. *Euthanasia* is defined in these studies as the termination of a person's life by someone other than the patient, upon the latter's explicit request. To get an accurate count of the total incidence of euthanasia one therefore has to include also cases in which euthanasia took place without explicit request, an important and troublesome problem to which I will return at a later point in this chapter.

TABLE 2.1   Frequency of Termination of Life as Proportion of All Deaths According to Year

	1990	1995	2001	2005
Euthanasia	1.7%	2.4%	2.6%	1.7%
Assisted suicide	0.2	0.2	0.2	0.1
Ending of life without explicit request	0.8	0.7	0.7	0.4
Total	2.7%	3.3%	3.5%	2.2%

Source: Agnes von der Heide, "End-of-Life Practices in the Netherlands Under the Euthanasia Act," *New England Journal of Medicine* 356 (2007): 1961.

The 1995–1996 interviews with the sample of 405 physicians provide information on the reasons why patients' request for euthanasia or PAS were granted or refused. Of the total of 9,700 requests received in 1995, 37% were granted; in about half of the remaining cases, the physician refused the request; and in the rest of the cases, either the patient died before a decision had been reached or he or she retracted the request. The most frequently mentioned reasons given by physicians for refusing the request for assisted death were that "suffering was not unbearable" (35%), that there existed alternative treatments (32%), that the patient was depressed or had other psychiatric symptoms (31%), or that the request "was not well considered" (19%).[29] Similar results are reported in a study of GPs carried out from April 2000 to December 2002, in which 44% of the explicit requests for euthanasia or PAS suicide were granted.[30]

The 1995–1996 interviews also revealed a lower rate of consultations in cases of refused requests. Thus, for example, whereas 79% of physicians who granted the request for assisted death consulted another physician, only 16% who refused a request sought a second opinion.[31] The law defines the consultant as the physician who should be consulted "with respect to the *intention* [my italics] to terminate a life on request or to assist in a suicide" (Article 1.d), and thus seems to cover both a considered as well as an executed assisted death. But perhaps, in those cases without consultation referred to in this study, the attending physician regarded these requests so obviously without merit that he saw no need for consulting a colleague.

We also have data on the characteristics of patients choosing euthanasia or PAS (Table 2.2). The patients making this choice tended to be

TABLE 2.2 Patients' Characteristics and Death Rate in Requested Cases of Euthanasia and Assisted Suicide (as Percentage of all Medical Decisions Concerning the End of Life [MDEL])

	1990	1995	2001	2005
Age (years)				
0–64	3.0%	4.6%	5.0%	3.5%
65–79	2.3	2.9	3.3	2.1
>80	1.0	1.2	1.4	0.8
Sex				
Male	2.1%	2.2%	3.1%	2.0%
Female	1.7	2.8	2.5	1.5
Underlying medical problem				
Cancer	4.4%	7.0%	7.4%	5.1%
Cardiovascular disease	0.5	0.3	0.4	0.3
Other or unknown	1.1	1.0	1.2	0.4

Source: Bregje D. Onwuteaka-Philipsen, et al., "Euthanasia and Other End-of-Life Decisions in the Netherlands in 1990, 1995, and 2001," *The Lancet* 362 (2003): 396-97.

younger, thus weakening the argument of critics who have alleged that, in a regime of accepted euthanasia, older people would be especially vulnerable and in danger of being euthanized. Those requesting euthanasia or PAS were more likely to be male than female, and most of them suffered from terminal cancer or other serious diseases, often with multiple complications.[32]

Most of the patients seeking assistance in dying are in the terminal stages of their illness. In the 1995 study, the estimated shortening of life was less than 24 hours in 17% of the cases and less than one week in 42% of the cases. Only 9% had a life expectancy of more than one month.[33] Studies for later years show similar figures.[34]

In line with findings from other countries, the most important reason for requesting euthanasia or PAS given in the 1990 study was loss of dignity (mentioned in 57% of cases), pain (46%), unworthy dying (46%), being dependent on others (33%), or tiredness of life (23%). In only 10 of 187 cases was intolerable pain the only reason for requesting aid in dying,[35] Similar results were obtained in a study of GPs carried out between April 2000 and December 2001, who were asked to describe the most recent requests for euthanasia or PAS they had received. In this study, patients mentioned pointless suffering as the reason for requesting euthanasia or

PAS in 75% of the cases, deterioration or loss of dignity in 69%, and pain only in 31% of all requests.[36] The fact that pain ranks rather low in the list of reasons for requesting aid in dying has an important bearing on the relationship of palliative care and euthanasia, a subject to which I will return.

Euthanasia and PAS are performed mainly by family physicians, who usually care for dying patients in their homes. During 2006, 88% of all such interventions were carried out by GPs, and 79% took place at the patients' home.[37] These doctors have known their charges for years and thus share their patients' tribulations. The assurance that their doctor will assist them if their suffering becomes unbearable has the result that about two-thirds of requests for euthanasia or PAS never actually lead to euthanasia or PAS.[38]

Euthanasia and PAS in the Netherlands enjoy wide popular support, and this support is related to the wish to have a dignified death and being able personally to decide end-of-life treatments.[39] A nationwide survey carried out in 2001–2002 showed that 82% of the population approved of physicians terminating life at the request of seriously ill patients, and 92% favored the legalization of assisted death carried out with due care.[40] The Dutch Roman Catholic Bishops are on record as opposing both euthanasia and PAS, which they regard as "neither permissible nor necessary."[41] However, in view of the wide support for euthanasia and PAS in the Dutch population, it is likely that many rank-and-file Dutch Catholics agree with the view of dissident theologian Hans Küng, who approves of the Dutch regime as representing a laudable middle-way between a libertarian individualism and the traditional Catholic rigorism.[42]

The great majority of the medical profession also considers euthanasia and PAS part of normal medical practice, aimed at protecting the dignity of the dying process, as is shown by the following figures (Table 2.3):

Sixteen percent of all deaths occur in nursing homes, where patients tend to be fragile and often incompetent, and where death takes place more frequently as a result of the withholding or withdrawal of treatment. A 2005 study of nursing home patients with dementia who died of pneumonia after doctors decided not to treat them with antibiotics revealed that, in 53% of these cases, there was an explicit intention to hasten death,

TABLE 2.3 Percentage of Physicians Participating in Euthanasia and Assisted Suicide

	1990	1995	2001
Performed it ever	54%	53%	57%
Performed it in previous 24 months	24	29	30
Never performed it but would be willing to do so under certain conditions	34	35	32
Would never perform it but would be willing to refer patient to another physician	8	9	10
Would never perform it nor refer patient	4	3	1

Source: Onwuteaka-Philipsen, et al., "Euthanasia and Other End-of-Life Decisions in the Netherlands," p. 397.

and in 41% of them, physicians reported taking into account the hastening of the end of life. Most of these patients were severely demented, and the acute illness was severe. The administration of lethal dosages, on the other hand, was rare.[43] According to data collected in 1994–1995, about a third (34%) of all psychogeriatric nursing homes had a written policy banning euthanasia or PAS.[44] Since most nursing homes are run by religious organization, it is possible that physicians in such homes are more reluctant to carry out euthanasia and PAS (Table 2.4). According to Griffiths's study, published in 1998, whereas physicians as a group granted about 40% of all requests for euthanasia and PAS, nursing home physicians complied with only 7% of all requests for euthanasia and 22% of those for assisted suicide. Many nursing homes voice the view that a permissive policy on assisted death would lead to fear and insecurity among their patients.[45]

TABLE 2.4 Type of Physician Performing Euthanasia and Assisted Suicide (as Percentage of all Medical Decisions Concerning the End of Life [MDEL])

	1990	1995	2001	2005
Family physician (GP)	3.1%	4.3%	5.8%	3.7%
Clinical specialist	1.4	1.8	1.8	0.5
Nursing home physician	0.1	0.3	0.4	0.2

Source: Onwuteaka-Philipsen, et al., "Euthanasia and Other End-of-Life Decisions in the Netherlands," p. 397; von der Heide et al., "End-of-Life Practices in the Netherlands Under the Euthanasia Act," p. 1962.

Euthanasia and PAS in the Netherlands are governed by rules and protocols adopted over time by various institutions and organizations involved in health care, and most of these rules predate the legalization law of 2002. For example, the Royal Dutch Pharmaceutical Association (KNMP) in 1987 issued guidelines on the preparation and use of drugs to be employed in euthanasia and PAS. On the basis of doctors' experiences, these guidelines were revised in 1994, 1998, and 2007. They include provisions such that (a) a pharmacist is free to decide whether or not to dispense drugs for euthanasia or assisted suicide; (b) the decision to dispense these drugs is to be taken after consultation with the involved physician, who is to give the pharmacist relevant information concerning the condition of the patient; and (c) the drug must be handed personally to the physician. A study of the implementation of these rules, based on data collected between 1994 and 1995, revealed some deviation from the guidelines. Unused drugs often were not returned, and pharmacy technicians, not supposed to be involved with the dispensing of these drugs, were found to handle drugs used in euthanasia and PAS.[46] As of this writing, I have not found more recent data that would show whether these irregularities have continued.

In 1992, the Foundation for Pharmaceutical Home Care Holland North developed a protocol concerning the performance by GPs of euthanasia and PAS in the home, where more than three-quarters of these interventions take place. Following these guidelines, the drug of choice for euthanasia is the oral administration of a barbiturate mixture to induce coma followed by a muscle relaxant given parenterally (by injection).[47]

The number of clinical complications that have occurred in the performance of euthanasia and PAS has been relatively small. According to a study published in 1997, the average time that elapsed between the administration of the drugs and death was 8 minutes (range 0–90 minutes). Three percent of GPs reported complications or unintended effects; another study found that problems occurred in 5% of the cases studied. These complications included spasm or myoclonus, and nausea and vomiting. The largest number of such problems was reported in cases of PAS: In many instances, patients had trouble using their hands or swallowing the oral medication. In 21 of 114 studied cases in which the original intention had been to provide assistance with suicide, the responsible physician decided to administer the lethal medication because of the anticipated failure of the assisted suicide. Hence, while the patient's final decision to end his or her life is more clearly articulated in PAS than in euthanasia—the voluntariness and the seriousness of the patient's request is proven by the fact that he or she has to perform the final act by him- or herself—the occurrence of complications probably is one of the reasons why the great majority of cases of assisted dying in the Netherlands involve euthanasia rather than PAS.[48]

Problems in the Practice of Euthanasia and Physician-assisted Suicide

Despite an extensive edifice of legal control and informal protocols governing the practice of euthanasia and PAS, many of them the result of professional self-regulation, several problem areas remain. It is to the credit of the Dutch medical profession, social scientists studying the practice of euthanasia and PAS in the Netherlands, and the various Dutch governments that these problems are recognized, are not swept under the rug, and that efforts to find solutions are taking place. Opinions may differ on how successful these efforts have been to date, but none can deny the impressive transparency that has been achieved. The vast majority of the numerous studies dealing with these unsolved problems have been published in English-language professional journals, so that the outside world has no difficulty in getting to know the true state of affairs with regard to the practice of euthanasia and PAS in the Netherlands—warts and all. In the discussion that follows, I take up the most important of these problem areas.

1. Failure to Report Cases of Euthanasia and Physician-assisted Suicide

Both before and after the legalization of euthanasia and PAS in 2002, enforcement of the rules that govern the practice of assisted death has depended to a crucial extent on the reports filed by physicians. When a physician reports a case of euthanasia or PAS as a natural death, there exists no way of finding out whether and to what extent he has adhered to the rules of due care. He can neither be disciplined by the authorities or the Medical Disciplinary Board for having violated the rules of reporting, nor can steps be taken to prevent him from repeating such illegal and unprofessional conduct in the future. Over the years, as we will see presently, the rate of reporting has improved considerably, but the problem of nonreporting has not yet been fully solved.

Until the legalization of euthanasia and PAS in 2002, even physicians following the rules of due care were still formally committing a criminal offense. Not surprisingly, in 1990, the rate of reporting was estimated to be 18%; in 1995, it was 41 percent, and in 2001, it was still only 54%. Despite the fact that, by 2001, a physician who conformed to the requirements of due care no longer faced a significant risk of prosecution, about half of all cases of euthanasia and PAS were still being reported to the authorities as natural deaths.[49] According to data published in 1998, physicians justified this widespread flouting of the reporting rules because of a combined desire to avoid the fuss of a judicial inquiry (52%), a wish to protect the family of the deceased from such an inquiry (29%), and the fear of prosecution, with its attendant costs in time, money, and emotional strain (24%).[50] The rate of reporting was also found to be influenced by the number of investigations undertaken by the public prosecutor in differing political climates, with doctors taking into account the concrete risk inherent in reporting cases of euthanasia and PAS at any particular point in time.[51]

Writing in 1997, the scholar John Griffiths and his co-authors surmised that even legalization of euthanasia and PAS would not increase the rate of reporting and that, in fact, it would make physicians less likely to do so. They reasoned that legalization would incorporate the requirements of due care in the criminal code, and that this would make prosecutors and judges act less flexibly in applying the codified rules to the varying circumstances of individual cases.[52] These fears turned out to be groundless. During the last few years, the rate of reporting has increased substantially, and by 2005, it reached 80%. A questionnaire study of physicians revealed that in 76% of the cases of nonreporting, doctors had not perceived their act as constituting the intentional ending of life but rather regarded it as the alleviation of symptoms or as palliative or terminal sedation with hastening of death as a possible side effect of the liberal use of opioids such as morphine.[53] The difference between these actions and euthanasia can be rather small and depends on what Timothy Quill appropriately has called "the protective umbrella of the double effect"— death is foreseen but not intended. "The potential for self-deception in such justifications is substantial."[54] Griffiths and his co-authors, who agree with Quill's appraisal, speak of the "constructability of the distinction between 'intentional termination'. . . and pain relief."[55] I will return to this issue in my discussion of palliative care.

The authors of the evaluation of the 2002 Euthanasia Act, published in 2007, concluded that the main reason for not reporting euthanasia and PAS was the belief of many doctors that their course of action did not constitute a life-terminating act. They had acted primarily to relieve the suffering of a dying patient rather than with the intention of avoiding the requirements of reporting and due care. Practically all of these cases involved the use of morphine, a drug that many physicians are less inclined to regard as life-shortening than the drugs typically used for euthanasia or PAS (barbiturates and/or neuromuscular relaxants). Still, they added, "this does not alter the fact that approximately 20% of all cases of life termination upon request are not reported."[56]

Many physicians are said to feel that aiding a patient to die is a private matter between doctor and patient, and that the intrusion of the state into this highly personal event therefore is inappropriate and insufficiently justified. The complexities of being a physician facing difficult decisions, they argue, cannot be handled satisfactorily by inflexible legal processes.[57] Existing data for 1994–1995 indeed show that most of the differences between reported and unreported cases of euthanasia and PAS did not involve the characteristics of patients (age, sex, diagnosis) but rather were related to procedural requirements. For example, consultation with another physician took place in 94% of reported, but only in 11% of unreported cases; a written report by the physician was filed in 97% versus 57% of unreported cases.[58]

Physicians who fail to report the performance of euthanasia cannot use the appropriate drugs because a request for these drugs will draw the suspicion of the pharmacist, who is required to inquire into the reasons for the request. This often has led doctors to resort to medications that are less than fully effective and that lead to complications.[59] Most importantly, adequate legal oversight over medical decisions involving matters of life and death is seen by many in the Netherlands as "the cornerstone of the formal accountability that is an essential condition of the social acceptability of the practice."[60] Opinions will probably continue to differ over to what extent the 2002 law has succeeded in reconciling rival considerations of privacy and accountability.

2. Ending Life Without Explicit Request of the Patient

The Remmelink Report of 1991 revealed that, in about 1,000 cases of euthanasia, the termination of life had taken place without the explicit request of the patient, and this discovery caused considerable consternation especially among non-Dutch critics. How could euthanasia in the Netherlands be considered voluntary if patients had not asked for assistance in dying? Since then, the frequency of such cases has declined from about 0.8% of all cases of death in 1990 to 0.4% in 2005 (Table 2.1), but the problem has not been eliminated. In 2005, in absolute numbers, there were still about 500 instances of life being ended without request (LAWER or Life-terminating Act Without Explicit Request [of the patient]).

Not all of these cases are morally problematic, although they do constitute a criminal offense. The 1991 data showed that 86% of the patients involved in these cases were considered incompetent and thus unable to participate in any meaningful way in the decision-making process. In 83% of the cases, it was no longer possible to communicate with the patient, and one of out three of these patients was permanently unconscious. The majority of these patients were in a terminal stage of cancer, accompanied by severe suffering. Eighty-seven percent were not expected to live more than one week, and more than 50% would have died within 24 hours.[61]

The 2005 questionnaire study evinced similar findings. The ending of life had not been discussed with patients in 10.4% of cases because these patients had been unconscious, or in 14.4% because the patient was incompetent owing to young age. There had been discussion of the act or a previous wish of the patient in 60% of the cases; in 80.9%, the ending of life had been discussed with relatives; and in 65.3%, the physician had discussed the decision with one or more colleagues. The desperate nature of these cases was brought out by the fact that, whereas in regular cases of euthanasia and PAS, life was shortened by less than one week for 44.8% of patients, in cases of LAWER this happened in almost double the number of cases (85.5%).[62] According to another study published in 2007, physicians estimated that these patients' lives had been shortened by less than one day in 44% of the cases.[63]

The following describes a case of LAWER that does not appear to be unjustified:

> An 81-year-old woman terminally ill with breast cancer and widespread bone metastases wanted to die at home. The general practitioner, who had known her for eight years, visited her regularly. The pain became more and more difficult to alleviate with opioids. The patient repeatedly mentioned that if her situation were to become degrading or the suffering unbearable "everything should be finished" but consciousness deteriorated rapidly, and this was never an explicit request. When the decubitus [bed sores] became extensive, and pain could no longer be relieved, the doctor, after discussions with a colleague, the home care nurse, and the patient's son, gave a very high dosage of opioids to shorten life. The patient died half an hour later. The doctor estimated that life was shortened by a week at most.[64]

In other known cases of LAWER, it is similarly reasonable to suppose that the person concerned would have wanted life to be ended if he had been able to express a wish, or that the termination of life indeed served the best interests of the dying patient. In other words, there is a difference between nonvoluntary euthanasia (without explicit request) and involuntary euthanasia (against the wishes of the patient). There is no evidence to show that Dutch law or practice tolerates the termination of life contrary to the will, expressed or presumed, of dying patients.[65]

And yet, some of these cases raise troubling questions. According to the 2001 study, 16% of patients whose lives were ended without request were fully competent, and there is no good explanation of why a request to die was not obtained.[66] A study of decisions to forego life-prolonging treatment (withholding or withdrawing treatment) published in 2000 showed that in some exceptional cases "physicians failed to discuss the nontreatment decision even with competent patients because they thought the decision was clearly the best for the patient."[67] In a 2007 study of doctors who had ended life without explicit consent, the percentage of those who acknowledged that they had done so because "the act was clearly in the best interest of the patient" or because "discussion would have done more harm than good" was found to be zero,[68] but it is questionable whether these figures can be considered reliable. The above-mentioned fact, that in 16% of such cases the patient put to death without his consent was fully competent, would seem to indicate that instances of paternalism and disregard for patient autonomy do occur in instances of euthanasia.

Practically no cases of LAWER are officially reported—two out of an estimated 1,000 cases in 1990, and three out of 900 in 1995.[69] This means, of course, that not only is there no transparency, but that the various control mechanisms are inoperative and the possibility of abuse cannot be ruled out. Many of these cases can best be described as mercy-killing, but, as one observer put it, it is "unlikely" that this was the case in all instances of LAWER.[70]

The number of physicians willing to perform euthanasia and PAS has remained more or less constant but the number of doctors prepared to end life without a patient's request has declined (Table 2.5).

The fact that the total number of LAWER cases, as well as the willingness of physicians to resort to this practice, has gone down refutes the existence of a slippery slope allegedly created by the legalization of euthanasia and PAS.[71] It also seems to indicate that Dutch doctors recognize the serious nature of this disregard of patient autonomy and self-determination that occurs in cases of LAWER. As Loes Pijnenborg and several other well-known students of the subject argued convincingly in an essay published in 1993, there will always be situations of terrible suffering of

TABLE 2.5 Percentage of Physicians Ending Life Without a Patient's Explicit Request

	1990	1995	2001
Performed it ever	27%	23%	13%
Performed it in previous 24 months	10	11	5
Never performed it but would be willing do so under certain conditions	32	32	16
Would never perform it	41	45	71

Source: Onwuteaka-Philipsen, et al. "Euthanasia and Other End-of-Life Decisions in the Netherlands," p. 397.

the kind in which a patient cannot give a clear judgment about the desired course of action. Hence, the challenge of LAWER is not likely to disappear, and some doctors will feel that in such exceptional situations LAWER can be justified. However, they added, there must be safeguards such as "optimal palliative care, discussion with relatives, a colleague, and nurses, reporting, and the absence of economic motives." The last of these requirements is probably the easiest to implement. The population of the Netherlands is fully insured for the costs of longstanding illness, and there is therefore no danger that doctors will be unduly influenced by the wishes of a family concerned about the financial cost of long-term care.[72]

Another Dutch expert, Gerritt van der Wal, has gone further. "The ultimate reason why termination of life without request is not permissible," he has argued, "is that in principle it will never be possible to draw a clear dividing line between unrequested and unwanted termination of life." However, even he has conceded that in "the rare extreme case" it may just "be necessary to do something which in essence is impermissible."[73]

3. Termination of Life in Pediatric Cases

As a result of rapid advances in neonatal medicine during the last two decades, pediatricians now encounter a growing number of newborns with serious disorders or deformities associated with severe and sustained suffering. In some premature babies, there is evidence of intracerebral hemorrhage causing severe brain damage. These cases confront doctors with extremely difficult decisions and represent some of the most difficult aspects of pediatric medicine. One way of dealing with these extraordinary cases has been the practice of not initiating or discontinuing treatment for such newborns, but the Euthanasia Law of 2002 created a new dimension to the problem. The law authorizes euthanasia or PAS for minors between the ages of 12 and 18 under strictly defined conditions of consent and involvement of parents. The question became whether, applying the rationale of the law, it would be acceptable deliberately to end the life of newborns and infants whose suffering cannot be adequately reduced, even though such children cannot express their own wishes. Pediatricians had been pondering this issue for some years.

From 1986 onward, a working group formed by the Pediatric Association of the Netherlands had discussed the various types of end-of-life
decisions arising in neonatal intensive care. In 1989, a preliminary report
focused on the withholding and withdrawal of treatment for patients who
might be able to survive with continuation of treatment. The issue of
intentionally ending life was left unresolved. The final report, "To do or
not to do? Boundaries of Medical Action in Neonatology," did address
this contentious issue and was approved by the general assembly of the
Pediatric Association of the Netherlands in November 1992.

The report distinguished three categories of end-of-life decisions for
newborns and infants: withholding life-sustaining treatment, withdrawing life-sustaining treatment, and intentional ending of life. According to
the report, the decision to withhold or withdraw treatment raised no ethical problem in cases of inevitable short-term death. Such cases represented medical decisions. However, if the baby had a chance of survival,
the future quality of life should be considered: "the mental and physical
burden of the infant's life, the infant's capacity to interact with his or her
environment, the self-sufficiency or dependency of the infant on caregivers and the health care system, and the expected life span. As these points
cannot be evaluated in a simple scoring system, the assessment has to be
made on the basis of the overall picture of the quality of the future existence of the individual patient." Parents and physicians were to share the
responsibility of this assessment, although the physician had to make the
final decision. The wishes of parents to continue treatment were to be
honored unless this would cause unbearable suffering to the child. "Before
taking end-of-life decisions, consultation of a team of at least two other
physicians and nurses is considered as mandatory."[74]

A minority of cases concerned newborns who are not dependent on
life-sustaining treatment but whose future quality of life has an extremely
poor prognosis. Examples are newborns with severe spina bifida and
hydrocephalus, for whom no successful surgery is possible. Dutch pediatricians, the report noted, had different views on the acceptability of
actively terminating life in such cases. Those who did agree to such a termination should not file a certificate of natural death.[75]

Two court cases, decided in the mid 1990s, provided some legal guidance for physicians, although the courts probably based their judgment in

great part on the evolving opinion of the medical profession. On March 22, 1993, obstetrician Henk Prins had terminated the life of a three-day-old severely defective baby with spina bifida, hydrocephalus, a spinal cord lesion, and brain damage. The medical team responsible for the baby, in consultation with the parents, had earlier decided to cease further medical treatment and to forego an operation for the baby's spina bifida, which was considered medically futile. With the baby suffering severe pain that could not effectively be treated, doctors and parents decided to end the baby's life with a lethal injection. Dr. Prins reported this act to the local coroner, and on April 26, 1995, he stood trial in the district court of Alkmaar for murder.

The Almaar court found the doctor not guilty of murder. It accepted Prins' defense of "justification because of necessity," sanctioned by the courts since the *Schoonheim* case of 1983. The doctor had faced an unavoidable conflict of duties between his duty to prolong life and his duty to alleviate unbearable suffering. This plea was accepted even though in this instance the patient (a three-day-old baby) had not made an explicit request for a termination of life. Dr. Prins' defense of necessity was accepted for the following four reasons: (a) the baby's suffering had been unbearable and hopeless, and there had not been another medically responsible way to alleviate it; (b) both the decision-making leading to the termination of life and the way it was carried out had satisfied the "requirements of careful practice"; (c) the doctor's behavior had been consistent with scientifically sound medical judgment and the norms of medical ethics; and (d) termination of life had taken place at the express and repeated request of the parents as legal representatives of the new-born baby.[76] The Amsterdam Court of Appeals, using similar reasoning, affirmed the holding of the District Court.

A second case concerned the general practitioner Kadijk, who, on April 26, 1994, had ended the life of a baby with trisomy-13, an incurable congenital disorder manifesting itself in deformities of the skull, face, and hands; malformation of the heart and kidney; and brain damage. The baby was given a life expectancy of six months to a year, but after 24 days at home the baby's suffering became worse and it became apparent that death was near. At that point, doctor and parents decided to end the baby's distress with a lethal injection. Dr. Kadijk reported the death of the child to the coroner as "not natural," and on November 13, 1995, he stood trial for murder. As in the *Prins* case, the district court of Groningen accepted the defense of "justification because of necessity" and acquitted Dr. Kadijk. The Leeuwarden Court of Appeals upheld the decision.[77]

In 1996, the Ministers of Health and Justice, acting jointly, established a consultative group to make proposals for an appropriate assessment and notification procedure for cases in which the life of a baby with a serious medical condition is deliberately ended. The group's report was issued in 1997 and, for the most part, endorsed the principles affirmed by the courts in the Prins and Kadijk cases. Still, doctors continued to find the prevailing practice very stressful, since, despite their conviction of having acted with due care, they continued to be under suspicion of murder. Some suggested that instead of coroners reporting such cases to the public prosecutor, it would be preferable to have them assessed by a committee with multidisciplinary (medical, legal, and ethical) expertise, analogous to the review committees recognized by the 2002 Euthanasia Act.[78]

In 2002, pediatricians at the University Medical Center Groningen, working in close cooperation with a district attorney, developed a protocol, known as the Groningen Protocol, that contained guidelines regarding euthanasia for newborns. By following this protocol, the authors suggested, doctors who ended the life of a newborn would provide the authorities all the information they needed for assessing cases of euthanasia for severely ill newborns and eliminate the need for interrogations by police officers. Complying with the protocol would not guarantee that the physician would not be prosecuted, but in the four cases in which the group had performed a deliberate life-ending procedure in a newborn— acting and reporting them in accordance with the protocol—none had resulted in a prosecution.[79]

The protocol stated that five medical requirements had to be fulfilled to justify the euthanasia of a newborn: The diagnosis and prognosis must be certain; hopeless and unbearable suffering must be present; the diagnosis, prognosis, and unbearable suffering must be confirmed by at least one independent doctor; both parents must give informed consent; and the procedure must be performed in accordance with accepted medical standards. The Protocol also contained a list of items of information that doctors should include in their report regarding the diagnosis and prognosis of the case, the consultation that had preceded the act of euthanasia, and a description of the actual procedure. Using this information, the authorities would be in a position to make an informed assessment.[80]

The co-authors of the Groningen Protocol, Dr. Eduard Verhagen, a physician and lawyer, and Dr. Pieter J.J. Sauer, a physician and doctor of philosophy, have expressed the hope that the use of the protocol will increase the willingness of doctors to report cases of euthanasia in desperately ill and badly deformed newborns. A national survey of neonatologists and pediatricians carried out in 1995 had shown that about 15–20 such cases occur annually, but an average of only three cases had been reported. That survey also revealed that 23% of pediatricians could conceive of carrying out euthanasia without the consultation of the parents.[81] The Groningen Protocol emphasizes the importance of reporting in order to prevent uncontrolled and unjustified instances of euthanasia, and insists that both parents must give their consent.

In June 2005, the Pediatric Association of the Netherlands accepted the Groningen Protocol as the national guideline, and later that year the governing Christian Democrats announced that they too would approve the Protocol. In November 2005, the Ministers of Justice and Health decided to set up a committee of experts to advise the public prosecutors on matters relating to the termination of neonatal life. The committee was to include specialists, such as neonatologists and child neurologists, as well as an ethicist. Terminating the life of a neonate would remain an offense, but, as in regard to euthanasia and PAS under the 2002 law, no prosecution would take place if the committee of experts concluded that the requirements embodied in the Groningen Protocol had been observed.[82]

Not everyone in the Dutch medical community has embraced the principles of the Groningen Protocol. The future viability of a severely handicapped newborn, it is argued by some, involves not a purely medical judgment and opens the door to an essentially subjective evaluation of quality of life. The decision of the parents carries the potential for bias because of the emotional, physical, and financial hardships they face in the long-term care of a severely disabled child.[83] Defenders of the protocol have insisted that the large majority of cases involved infants for whom life-sustaining treatment had been foregone previously and where all possible palliative measures had been exhausted.[84] As of this writing, we have no data on the rate of reporting or other aspects of the practice of euthanasia for newborns since the adoption of the Groningen Protocol.

4. Assisted Death for Patients with Mental Suffering

Article 2 of the Euthanasia Act of 2002 requires that the request of a patient for assisted death be "voluntary and well-considered," and that would seem to call into question the eligibility of psychiatric patients whose competence to make such a request is commonly considered impaired by the mental illness with which they are afflicted. Problems may also arise in establishing that such a patient's suffering is "unbearable," another requirement of the Act. And yet, while requests for assisted death by psychiatric patients are rarely granted (according to 2000–2001 data, less than 1% of all cases of euthanasia and PAS)[85], both Dutch medical professional organizations and the courts for some time have taken the position that unbearable mental suffering can, in exceptional cases, justify the termination of life. The 2007 annual report of the Regional Euthanasia Review Committees reported six cases of euthanasia for patients with incipient dementia who nevertheless had a clear awareness of their disease and therefore were held able to give an informed consent.[86]

In 1985, the Dutch Medical Association appointed a Commission on the Acceptability of Medical Behavior That Shortens Life (CAL). The last of the four reports issued by this commission dealt with patients unable or not competent to request euthanasia, including persons suffering from mental illness. Entitled "Assistance with Suicide in Psychiatric Practice" (CAL 4), this report was published in November 1993. CAL 4 rejected the position that all psychiatric patients are incompetent to ask for assisted death. The patient's actual competence, not the psychiatric disorder, should be decisive. Certain treatable psychiatric conditions may give rise to temporary suicidal wishes or attempts. Doctors, the report argued, must distinguish between "a request that is really meant as such, and one that may well be the symptom of some temporary or treatable condition." In cases in which no successful treatment was possible, it was meaningless to "interpret the patient's wish for death as the result of a psychiatric condition."[87]

A report on assistance with suicide for psychiatric patients issued by the Dutch Association for Psychiatry (NVP) in 1997 took a similar position. It too rejected the idea that all psychiatric patients lack the normal human capacity for a well-considered request for assistance in dying. On the other hand, the report stressed that in these kinds of cases the patient's request had to be based on an "enduring desire for the end of life." This meant that the request must be made "over a period of *at least several months*, in a well-considered way, repeatedly, and in the presence of others."[88] Both reports insisted that because of the special susceptibility of psychiatric patients to suggestion and influence, and the danger that the psychiatrist, too, may be influenced in his judgment by unconscious motives, there should be consultation with one, and in difficult cases more than one, independent psychiatrist (or other doctor). The consultants must examine the patient themselves.[89] There is general agreement that in cases of nonsomatic suffering, special procedural safeguards are necessary.

Meanwhile, in 1994, the issue of assisted death for psychiatric patients had reached the Supreme Court. The case concerned Ms. B., a 50-year-old woman, who over the course of several years had undergone a series of traumatic experiences, including the loss of two sons, that had left her severely depressed and unwilling to go on living. Psychiatric treatment had had little effect, she had made one serious suicide attempt, and had refused further therapy. Her psychiatrist, Dr. Boudlwijn Chabot, consulted seven other physicians, five of whom supported the request for PAS, although none of them actually saw or examined the patient. On September 28, 1991, Dr. Chabot provided Ms. B. with a lethal drug, which she consumed in the presence of himself, a GP, and a friend. She died shortly thereafter, and Chabot reported her death to the coroner as an assisted suicide.[90]

The district court of Assen and the Court of Appeals, Leeuwarden, accepted Dr. Chabot's plea of "justification because of necessity," and found the psychiatrist not guilty. On appeal, the Supreme Court agreed with the holding of the Court of Appeals "that the wish to die of a person whose suffering is psychic can be based on an autonomous judgment." In principle, therefore, assistance in dying for psychiatric patients was not ·necessarily ruled out. However, the court insisted, in cases of patients who were not in a terminal phase of a somatic illness, the physician involved had to act with the utmost carefulness. Dr. Chabot had not acted in this way, and the court therefore found insufficient evidence to support the defense of necessity. There was no statement from an independent medical expert who had personally examined the patient. In cases of suffering that is psychic rather than somatic, the court ruled, such evidence was essential. It was not simply a procedural rule but a condition of the justification of necessity. The judgment of the independent consultant should cover the seriousness of the suffering and the prospects for improvement, alternatives to assistance with suicide, and the question whether the patient's request was voluntary and well-considered, "without [the patient's] competence being influenced by his sickness or condition." Dr. Chabot therefore was found guilty of the offense of assistance with suicide, although the court imposed no punishment.[91]

Following the Supreme Court's decision in the *Chabot* case, the Ministers of Health and Justice announced a revision of prosecutorial guidelines to conform to the Court's ruling, and 11 of 15 pending prosecutions involving nonterminal psychiatric patients were dropped. The Medical Inspectorate for Public Mental Health drew its own view of the case and filed a complaint against Dr. Chabot with the Medical Disciplinary Board. Although the Board agreed with the ruling of the Supreme Court that assisted suicide can be justified for patients whose suffering does not have a somatic base and who are not in a terminal condition, it did find that Dr. Chabot had not acted according to accepted professional standards and reprimanded him.[92]

Another case raising somewhat similar issues arose several years later. Edward Brongersma was an 86-year-old single man, obsessed with his physical decline and existential suffering, who had concluded that his life had become meaningless; he repeatedly asked his physician, Dr. Philip Sutorius, to help him die. Two other doctors consulted by Dr. Sutorius—a family physician and a psychiatrist—confirmed the man's hopeless suffering, although they found no serious somatic or psychiatric illness. On April 22, 1998, Dr. Sutorius assisted Mr. Brongersma to commit suicide, and reported it to the authorities.[93]

Dr. Sutorius was indicted for having assisted a suicide, but after hearing from three medical experts that Brongersma had indeed been suffering unbearably and that there existed no appropriate medical treatment for his condition, the District Court of Haarlem acquitted the doctor. The public prosecutor, seeking to set "a principled boundary" regarding end-of-life decisions for people without a medical illness, appealed this verdict, and in May 2001, the Court of Appeal in Amsterdam agreed to hear the case. The decision of this court, which found Sutorius guilty of not adhering to the criteria of due care, relied heavily on the testimony of two experts on medical law and the care of the chronically ill. These experts had argued that a doctor's role should be limited to matters within the medical domain, and that the problem of elderly people who no longer wanted to live was a social rather than a medical problem. The court also questioned the lower court's stipulation that the situation had been "without prospect of relief," suggesting that Sutorius had failed to explore other means of relieving Brongersma's life fatigue. However, since Dr. Sutorius, in the court's view, had acted with integrity and good faith, no punishment was imposed. The Supreme Court confirmed this ruling on December 24, 2002.[94]

In the wake of the *Brongersma* case, the Royal Dutch Medical Association appointed a commission of inquiry, and in December 2004, the commission, headed by Professor of Psychology J.H. Dijkhuis, issued its report, "Searching for Norms for Physician Intervention When Help Is Requested to End Life in Case of Emotional Suffering." The Dijkhuis commission noted that the number of such requests is very low, and that the Dutch medical profession had not developed a professional consensus with regard to the problem of existential suffering without an incurable medical disease. After reviewing various options, the commission recommended that life fatigue in principle be accepted as a valid reason for assisted death, leaving it up to individual physicians how to respond to such requests. It also suggested that procedural guidelines be developed on how to evaluate this special kind of suffering. The commission pointed out that the Euthanasia law of 2002 required the presence of suffering that was "lasting and unbearable" (Article 2.1.b), but did not prescribe how this suffering should be assessed.[95]

The Djkhuis commission report is unlikely to end the debate within the medical profession about its proper role in dealing with existential suffering. Relying on the principles of respect for autonomy and beneficence, some argue that doctors have a duty to respect their patients' autonomous preferences and that they must act in the interests of patients whose suffering is unbearable, no matter what the source of this suffering. They should also take into account the risk of a violent suicide if the request for assisted death is denied. Others fear that such an expansion of the medical domain may undermine the legitimacy of voluntary euthanasia in cases of more obvious medical suffering and may reinforce the image of the doctor as "hangman." Moreover, once the suffering elderly are brought into the reach of the euthanasia law, what is to prevent the extension of such assisted death for others similarly tired of life and also suffering severely?[96]

Still others, including the Dutch Association for Voluntary Euthanasia, have expressed the fear of a new kind of "ageism" that may lead to the rejection of requests for euthanasia by the elderly simply because they express their death wish less clearly and forcefully, and their request therefore is taken less seriously. Sometimes a formerly expressed death wish is eventually not honored because the patient becomes confused and depressed. At times, doctors are less cooperative because they want to prevent any suspicion that the lives of older people are endangered. It is a fact, mentioned earlier, that the percentage of people dying of euthanasia is lower among those above the age of 80 than among younger patients, and a study by Ilinka Haverkate published in 2001 reported that euthanasia is more often denied to older than to younger people. None of these data are very conclusive as to cause and effect, and further research on this problem is needed.[97]

To spare the elderly situations of physical deterioration, dependency, loneliness, confinement to a nursing home, or the prospect of dementia, the suggestion has been made that people above a certain age be given the right of "rational suicide." In 1991, Huib Drion, a retired chairman of the Dutch Supreme Court, published an article entitled "The Self-desired End of Elderly People" in a popular Dutch newspaper which began: "I don't believe there is any doubt that many elderly people would be comforted and relieved if they were able to obtain a means to leave life in an acceptable way at the moment that suits them." Drion suggested that doctors make a pill available to all people above the age of 75 that would give these elderly a right of death at the time of their choosing. The idea of what became known as "Drion's Pill" created considerable discussion, but according to 2001–20002 data, a majority of doctors do not favor this plan. Fifty-six percent opposed the scheme, 25% were in favor, and 19% had no opinion.[98] The Dutch Association for Voluntary Euthanasia (NVVE), on the other hand, is said to have voted in March 2002 in favor of working for the free distribution of medications for suicide.[99]

Dutch psychiatrists take a cautious view of assisted death for patients with mental problems. A survey of psychiatrists conducted in 1996 showed that 37% of respondents had at least once received an explicit and persistent request for PAS from a patient, but only 2% had actually once assisted in such a suicide. In many of these cases, there was both a mental disorder as well as a serious physical illness, often in a terminal phase. The most frequently given reasons for not acting on such a request from a mental patient was the belief that the patient had a treatable mental disorder, opposition in principle to assisting in suicide, and doubts that the patient's suffering was unbearable or hopeless.[100] Predictions of outcome for individual psychiatric patients are not very reliable, as is shown by the poor success psychiatrists have in predicting suicide.[101] It is well known that the death wish of very ill patients is often associated with clinical depression, and while many instances of depression are indeed well-justified by the wretched condition of a severely suffering person, it is not clear at what point depression precludes rational decision making. Not surprisingly, in a survey published in 2005, a finding that the patient requesting assistance in dying was not fully competent was one of the main reasons given by GPs for refusing such assistance.[102]

A study at the University Center Utrecht of cancer patients with an estimated life expectancy of three months or less, who knew that their cancer was untreatable, found that a fifth of these patients had made an explicit request for euthanasia. Among these terminal patients, those with a depressed mood had requested assisted death four times as often as those without such a condition.[103] And yet, although primary care physicians often find it difficult to spot the presence of depression and there exists therefore a definite risk of such a physician misjudging a patient's competency, few consult a psychiatrist. According to a study published in 2004, the annual number of such psychiatric consultations was estimated to be no more than 4% of all requests for PAS.[104]

The authors of the Utrecht study suggested that "physicians consult a psychiatrist whenever they have doubts about whether the depressed mood of a patient affects his or her decision-making ability," but they were unsure about making such a consultation mandatory (sometimes called a "psychiatric filter"). There was the risk of further burdening terminally ill patients, especially since the value of such a consultation was not clearly established. An earlier study has shown that a standard psychiatric evaluation changed the policy of the primary care physician in only 9% of the cases. The author of that study questioned the wisdom of making psychiatrists the final gatekeepers of assisted death.[105] In a discussion, released in 2001, of the pending euthanasia legislation by the Dutch Foreign Ministry, it was stated that in cases of mental illness two doctors should be consulted, at least one of them a psychiatrist,[106] but this provision did not make it into the final bill.

The answer to the question whether psychiatric examinations should be made mandatory depends in part on the extent to which the presence of depression is seen to affect the decision-making ability of sick persons. There are therapy-resistant depressed patients, whose suffering is perpetual and unbearable, who in relatively good periods can rationally assess their future alternatives. A.J.F.M. Kerkhof, the author of the study that drew attention to these kinds of cases, nevertheless came out in favor of a psychological evaluation. A request for suicide, he pointed out, can mean different things. It can be a request for actual assistance to die or a request for help in living. The true meaning of the request may not even be clear to the patient. "A second opinion should therefore always be given by a psychiatrist, psychologist, or mental health care worker." The availability of assisted suicide in exceptional circumstances, Kerkhof insisted, is not in conflict with the ideal of preventing suicide. "The availability of this choice, among many other things, contributes to early identification of suicide risk and improved mental health care delivery for the majority of (nonexceptional) cases in which there is still a treatment option."[107] There is general agreement that further research into the circumstances that may require a psychiatric examination is needed.

Another area of disagreement concerns the use of advance directives. Article 2.2 of the Euthanasia Act allows doctors to act on requests for assisted death from a person who "is no longer capable of expressing his will, but prior to reaching this condition was deemed to have a reasonable understanding of his interests and has made a written statement containing a request for termination of life." The law also requires that the requirements of due care, *mutatis mutandis,* be fulfilled, but questions have been raised whether this indeed possible. For example, if a person has become comatose, can his suffering be considered "unbearable" (Article 2.1.b)?[108] It is not clear whether a severely demented patient is indeed "suffering" from the dementia. Will a doctor know enough about the decision-making process that led to the signing of the advance directive, perhaps years earlier, to be sure that "the request by the patient was voluntary and well-considered" (Article 2.1.a)? Given the uncertainties inherent in psychiatric diagnosis and prognosis, can the doctor who has to decide *when* to carry out the patient's advance request be sure that there exists "no other reasonable solution for the situation [of the patient]" (Article 2.1.d)? Can the consulting physician who has to examine an incompetent patient, while most likely unable to communicate with him or her, be able to determine and certify that "the requirements of due care, referred to in parts a–d" (Article 2.2.e) have been met?[109]

Solutions may be found to some or all of these challenges, but it remains that, under these circumstances of uncertain knowledge, a doctor's burden in making such an irreversible decision may simply be too great. As of this writing, no data are available on the frequency of euthanasia and PAS on the basis of an advance directive.

5. *Can Palliative Care Eliminate the Need for Assisted Death?*

Palliative care is defined as "the study and management of patients with active, progressive, far-advanced disease for whom the prognosis is limited and the focus of care is quality of life."[110] Palliative care began as part of the modern hospice movement that originated in 1967, with the foundation of St. Christopher's Hospice in southeast London by Dame Cicely Saunders. The ideals of hospice and palliative care have since spread to all corners of the world. The basic aim of palliative care is to alleviate suffering for terminal patients. In the words of one proponent:

> In palliative care, nothing is undertaken to postpone unnecessarily or intentionally to hasten death. Life-prolonging treatment, which is potentially harmful for the well-being of terminal patients and which can make

the acceptance of their situation more difficult, is deemed futile. Intentionally hastening death is regarded as dangerous and unnecessary since patients' requests for euthanasia are often ambivalent and preventable in the context of good palliative care.[111]

And yet, although palliative care in most instances is indeed able to provide terminal patients with relative comfort and a tolerably "good death," it is generally acknowledged that in some few cases of dying suffering is unbearable and irreversible, and physicians are unable to palliate the agony of these patients. Symptoms such as feelings of suffocation, nausea, and anxiety appear particularly difficult to control.[112] Moreover, as a survey published in 2006 again confirmed, many patients do not want to live to the bitter end, even if their pain and suffering can be controlled. They fear a loss of dignity during a prolonged dying process and do not want to burden their families with terminal care. They want to decide for themselves when and how to die, and wish to be remembered by their families the way they were when they were more or less healthy. This sentiment appears to be especially strong in the Netherlands,[113] and it therefore is likely that palliative care and assisted death will continue to coexist rather than exclude each other.

All over the Western world, recognition of the importance of palliative care has been a relatively late development, and this was especially the case in the Netherlands. Health care there is characterized by a strong emphasis on primary care delivered in the patient's home. General practitioners and nurses have always been attentive to the needs of their charges on a 24-hour basis, and have given high priority to care for the dying. Hence, while most European countries began to develop specialist palliative care services in the early 1980s, such services came to the Netherlands only in the 1990s. The Johannes Hospice in Vleuten opened in 1991, the Rozenheuvel hospice near Arnhem—eventually to become internationally known for its outstanding work—was started in 1994.[114] Most of the other hospices that followed are run by volunteers who also visit patients in their homes. They are known as "low-care hospices" or "almost-at-home-homes"; the medical care of their patients remains the responsibility of the GP treating these patients.

By 2005, there were also 15 so-called high-care hospices, which have on staff a physician specialized in palliative care. These hospices do not allow euthanasia on their premises, and indeed seek to demonstrate that good palliative care makes euthanasia unnecessary.[115] Although 25% of the 517 patients admitted to the Hospice Rozenheuvel between 1994 and 1995 stated upon admission that they wanted euthanasia when their suffering became unbearable, only two persisted in this wish and were eventually transferred to a hospital to receive euthanasia.[116] It is not clear whether these figures prove that good palliative care makes euthanasia unnecessary. Some have suggested that more patients in such a hospice might ask for euthanasia, "but because of the warm attention given to them by so many, and because they know their caregivers are opponents of euthanasia, they do not dare to."[117]

Palliative care developed in the Netherlands at a time when euthanasia and PAS had already been accepted by the majority of the population, and this has given rise to the charge that the late arrival of palliative care was the result of physicians having ready recourse to easier, yet more lethal, methods of dealing with the travail of dying.[118] The 2001 survey of the euthanasia program revealed that 41% of Dutch physicians agreed with the statement that preoccupation with assisted death had led to the neglect of other methods to ease the suffering of the dying, and 30% thought that the quality of palliative care in the Netherlands left much to be desired.[119] Still, whatever neglect may have existed, today it is generally recognized that, since the mid 1990s, Dutch palliative care has taken giant steps forward. By that time, all political parties had begun to realize that a responsible policy regarding euthanasia and PAS would be possible only in the context of a well-developed system of palliative care.[120]

In 1996, the government promised to make 250,000 guilders ($US120,000) available for the development of palliative care, and within a year this sum was raised to 35,000,000 guilders ($US17,000,000). In 1997, the first local Palliative Care Consultation Team was established and, by March 2002, there were 20 such teams covering two-thirds of the country. The consultants to these teams are medical specialists (oncologists, radiotherapists, and anesthesiologists) and nurses from hospices or oncology departments, all with extra expertise in palliative care. They are supported by psychologists, social workers, members of the clergy (to provide pastoral care), and pharmacists. These teams can be consulted by all professionals involved in palliative care by phone or, when requested by a caregiver, a patient can by visited by a consultant. These teams have enhanced GP competence in the field of palliative care: According to a survey published in 2004, 65% of GPs felt that the quality of their care of the dying had improved.[121]

In 1998, a national palliative care program was launched to stimulate education and research in palliative care, and six Centers for the Development of Palliative Care (COPZs) were established at university hospitals to enhance coordination in care giving, develop educational modules, and increase expertise, as well as to carry out research. The COPZs, financially supported by the government until 2002, directed multidisciplinary regional consulting teams, and by 2000, these teams were estimated to be accessible to care workers providing care to 43% of the Dutch population. All hospitals now have special pain management teams. A National Support Center for Palliative Care, Agora, financed by the government, monitors palliative care and submits quarterly and yearly reports to the ministry of health. In 2005, recognizing the uniqueness of palliative care for children, Agora established the Dutch Foundation for Palliative Care for Children and, as of 2006, there exist four children's hospices providing terminal and respite care.[122]

Palliative care in the Netherlands is integrated into the existing health care infrastructure along with nursing homes, hospitals and home care services. By 2002, 37 nursing homes, 26 retirement homes, and three hospitals had a hospice unit, but these units handle only a relatively small number of deaths. A government report issued in 2003 showed that of the approximately 40,000 persons annually dying of cancer, 65% die at home, over 25% in a hospital, about 6% in a nursing or retirement home, but less than 1% in a hospice facility. Most terminally ill patients in the Netherlands prefer to die at home in the care of their family physician, and the organization of palliative care tries to accommodate this wish.[123]

During the last ten years, palliative care in the Netherlands has made great progress. Elsewhere, a survey of physicians in specialties that frequently attend dying patients was carried out in late 2002, in Australia and Europe. This survey revealed that about half of all of these doctors had received some formal training in palliative care. Among Dutch doctors, 78% had gone through such training, a ratio far above that of any other country.[124] Yet, it is generally agreed that more can and should be done. Palliative care is still not part of all medical and nursing curricula, and many GPs are probably not yet sufficiently trained in this field, which is so important for quality end-of-life care and the prevention of mistakes. According to 2001 data, 36% of physicians agreed with the statement that because of insufficient knowledge of palliative care doctors frequently are not able to judge whether alternatives exist for alleviating the suffering of terminal patients.[125] The SCEN program is popular and widely used, but there is no obligation for GPs to consult SCEN physicians who have the expertise to assess possible palliative alternatives.[126]

Greater attention to and improvements in palliative care may account for the decline in the number of cases of euthanasia and PAS between 2001 and 2005, noted earlier in this chapter (Table 2.1), and the increased use of continuous deep sedation (also called *terminal sedation,* because it induces unconsciousness that lasts until the patient's death) that was involved in 22.2% of all deaths by 2003.[127] In 2001, 5.6% of all MDELs involved continuous deep sedation, whereas by 2005, the rate had risen to 7.1% of all such cases.[128] The rate of all MDELs involving euthanasia and PAS during this period decreased from 5.0% to 3.5%. Agnes van der Heide and her co-authors, who reported this development, note that "Dutch physicians have been found to consider high-quality end-of-life care as an alternative to euthanasia or assisted suicide, at least in some cases. In our study, we found that euthanasia and assisted suicide were to some extent replaced by continuous deep sedation. . . . Physicians also sometimes administer sedatives when they have the explicit intention of hastening death, such that sedation and euthanasia are not mutually exclusive in all cases."[129]

In August 2003, the attorney general proposed that terminal sedation be covered by the same legal controls as euthanasia, but this proposition was not adopted. The government accepted the arguments of the KNMG that terminal sedation, even when accompanied by the withdrawal of artificial feeding and hydration, constituted normal medical treatment and was therefore different from euthanasia.[130] It is known that in the vast majority of cases in which terminal sedation becomes an option, patients will have stopped eating and drinking by themselves, so that the withholding of food and drink does not constitute an ethical problem. Moreover, terminal sedation typically is used when the death of the patient is imminent. One study showed that in 75% of these cases, death was expected within a week. It is not known whether the substitution of terminal sedation for euthanasia is always in accordance with the wishes of the patient. According to 2005 data, in 9% of the cases, the decision to use continuous deep sedation was preceded by a request for euthanasia or PAS that had been denied.[131]

A relatively small minority of Dutch physicians, while recognizing that the difference between euthanasia and terminal sedation is small, nevertheless insists that a crucial borderline exists between administering barbiturates and euthanasia. Many of these doctors are associated with the high-care hospices, the vast majority of which (14 out of 15) are based on Christian values. Several years ago, the debate over how best to meet the needs of patients whose suffering does not respond to palliative care became quite heated. In one such exchange, a nursing home doctor charged hospice physicians who deny that high doses of morphine amount to euthanasia with extreme hypocrisy. Physicians who accepted the legitimacy of euthanasia felt that opponents of euthanasia unfairly criticized the quality of their palliative care. They insisted that even the best palliative care cannot put an end to all request for euthanasia or PAS, a point of view not necessarily rejected by all proponents of palliative care. Differences of opinion also developed over the best place to provide palliative care. Caregivers in nursing homes maintained that they had the longest experience in the field of palliative care, whereas physicians associated with hospices often found fault with the quality of palliative care given in regular health care institutions. Data on the quality of palliative care are difficult to find, and these discussions therefore will probably continue, albeit not necessarily in a highly aggressive form. Good palliative care probably can be provided in a variety of institutions.[132]

National organizations such as Agora and the Dutch Association for Palliative Care, established in 1996, have not taken sides in these debates, and, respecting the plurality of views among their members, have remained neutral. The goal of improving palliative care, they feel, is shared by all involved. On the other hand, the Dutch Right to Die Association (NVVE), founded in 1973 and listing more than 100,000 members, has expressed concern over what it sees as an increased preference of doctors for palliative care over euthanasia, perceiving this trend as a challenge to patient autonomy.[133]

Among professional caregivers, there appears to be growing recognition that many cases of both euthanasia and terminal sedation involve ethical dilemmas that defy an easy solution. In many instances, the distinction between euthanasia and symptom alleviation represents a "gray area," and doctors who administer high doses of a pain reliever do not always find it easy to interpret their own motives. An anthropologist who studied cases of euthanasia and PAS in a Dutch 400-bed teaching hospital found that "it is extremely difficult to establish what 'taking into account the probability or the certainty that the patient's death would thereby be hastened' and 'the partly intended hastening of the patient's death' mean. . . . Complex situations, motives, and decisions become simpler and more consistent when they are reconstructed afterward." At the time when a decision has to be made, the doctor's intentions may be quite equivocal.[134]

An increasing number of physicians have realized that greater familiarity with palliative care has improved their ability to decide whether the suffering of dying patients is indeed hopeless and unbearable, and more of them now resort to euthanasia or PAS only when no other alternatives are available. At the same time, in 2001, almost two-thirds (61%) of all doctors expressed the view that adequate treatment of pain and terminal care did not make euthanasia redundant.[135]

It may well be that in the years before the Dutch palliative care system reached its present well-developed state, lives were terminated because doctors had inadequate familiarity with palliative alternatives. There are those who think that "since palliative care is still developing it is safe to say that this problematic practice has not yet been abolished."[136] Yet this appraisal, while not completely invalid, may be unduly pessimistic. Even the best-trained physicians are known to make mistakes, and error-free medical practice is impossible. It would seem to be far more likely that, in view of the great strides made by Dutch palliative care during the last decade, the great majority of those suffering terminal patients who still insist on euthanasia or PAS do so for valid personal reasons and not because of the inadequacy of their terminal care and the unavailability of other remedies.[137]

The Dutch Regime of Euthanasia and Physician-assisted Suicide Assessed

In line with the purpose of this book, my aim in the last section of this chapter is not to present a full-fledged personal assessment of the Dutch practice of euthanasia and PAS. Rather, I want to look briefly at some of the arguments made by those who have written critically about this regime, and ascertain to what extent their arguments may be supported or contradicted by the actual practice of euthanasia and PAS described herein. It is worth remembering again the insight of Dutch scholar Johannes J.M. Delden that "facts will not settle a moral debate," but one cannot do ethics properly unless one knows the facts.[138] Many contenders in this highly charged controversy have at times disregarded this important principle.

The numerous studies undertaken by Dutch doctors and social scientists of the Netherlands' euthanasia and PAS regime have focused on specific problems, such as the failure to comply with reporting requirements, the problem of advance directives, or the ending of life without specific consent. These criticisms have been advanced to overcome what are conceded to be serious faults, and to explore remedies. By contrast, some foreign critics cite these shortcomings to buttress their conclusion that the entire system is basically flawed and poses a threat to important human values.

"Virtually every guideline established by the Dutch to regulate euthanasia has been modified or violated with impunity," wrote American psychiatrist Herbert Hendin in 1997. The system, he stated, is "basically out of control."[139] In an essay published five years later, but relying for the most part on data from the 1990 and 1995 surveys, Hendin repeated this harsh judgment. "The extension of euthanasia to more patients has been associated with the inability to regulate the process within established rules. Virtually every guideline set up by the Dutch—a voluntary, well-considered, persistent request; intolerable suffering that cannot be relieved; formal consultation with a colleague; and reporting of cases—has failed to protect patients or has been modified or violated." The Dutch effort to regulate euthanasia and PAS, Hendin concluded, has shown that "these practices defy adequate regulation. Given legal sanction, euthanasia, intended originally for the exceptional case, has become an accepted way of dealing with serious or terminal illness in the Netherlands. In the process, palliative care is one of the casualties, while hospice care lags behind that of other countries." Hendin found the Netherlands caught on a "slippery slope"—"the gradual extension of assisted suicide to widening groups of patients after it is legally permitted for patients designated as terminally ill." This included the chronically ill and even those afflicted with psychological distress.[140]

In a book published in 2002 (but, as in the case of Hendin, relying on data from the 1990 and 1995 surveys), British ethicist John Keown voiced the same wholesale condemnation of the Dutch practice of euthanasia and PAS. The guidelines for the regulation of euthanasia and PAS, he argued, were elastic and imprecise and had "conspicuously failed" in ensuring effective control. Dutch representations to the contrary, Keown maintained, "the reality is that guidelines have been widely breached and with effective impunity. . . . The undeniable want of effective control lends strong support to the empirical slippery slope argument."[141]

The first problem with the harshly negative conclusions reached by Hendin and Keown is that they rely on outdated data.[142] To use just one important example, the rate of reporting since 1995 has increased from 41% to 80%, and in cases of physicians who use drugs typically used for euthanasia and PAS (barbiturates and/or muscle relaxants), the percentage of reported cases is now estimated to be 99%. As we have seen, in recent years, nonreporting cases are largely connected to the use morphine as a means of life termination, which many physicians are less inclined to regard as life-shortening.[143] The Dutch authors who reported these data themselves acknowledged that a nonreporting rate of 20% was still too high and undercut the achievement of full transparency envisaged by the 2002 law. However, this notable improvement in the rate of reporting surely does not prove the existence of a slippery slope. The same goes for the impressive improvements in palliative care detailed earlier. Among European physicians, Dutch doctors are now considered the best-trained in this branch of medicine, so vital in finding alternatives to euthanasia and PAS.

The charge made by Hendin and Keown that the guidelines for due care in the practice of euthanasia and PAS can be violated with impunity and that therefore no effective control exists is in part related to the reliance of the Dutch regime on self-reporting and on the incomplete rate of reporting. It is true that what is not known cannot be restrained or disciplined. Yet, as we have seen, doctors who failed to report their terminal care as euthanasia did so primarily because of their belief that they had acted to relieve the suffering of a dying patient, rather than with the intention of avoiding the requirements of reporting and due care. Most of the cases that required action by the five regional review committees appeared to concern procedural lapses rather than substantive, serious violations of the law.

During 2003, 2004, and 2005, the review committees asked for further information from the physician or the consultant in 120 cases (6% of the about 2,000 reported cases of euthanasia and PAS) because of uncertainty or doubt regarding one or more of the requirements of due care. They issued a verdict of noncompliance in 15 of these cases and referred them to the judicial authorities.[144] One Dutch critic, Henk ten Have, has suggested that the committees have insufficient time to review each of these many cases in depth.[145] Others maintain that the low rate of serious violations indicates increased knowledge on the part of doctors on how to act properly in regard to requests for euthanasia or PAS.[146] The work of the review committees has also been praised for communicating the reasoning behind the committees' decisions to the medical community and thus exercising an important educational role.[147] Further research on the work of the review committees may throw additional light on these issues.

The American critic Neil Gorsuch has argued that some of the published Dutch survey data intentionally minimize the extent to which deaths are caused by the withdrawal or withholding of treatment without the explicit consent of the patient.[148] It is true, as Griffiths and his co-authors acknowledged in their study published in 1998, that the ending of life as a result of abandoning or withdrawing life-prolonging treatment or through the use of deep sedation involves a far larger number of patients than do instances of euthanasia and PAS. As we have seen, in many of these cases, treatment is ended without the patient's request because he or she is unconscious or otherwise unable to make his or her wishes known.[149] However, not only are data on these practices in the Netherlands fully available, but it is important to recognize that these same actions take place in other countries. In fact, according to a study published in 2007, ending the life of patients without their specific request took place at the same or occasionally even higher rates in some other societies. For example, in Belgium, the rate was 3.2% of all deaths in 1998 and 1.5% in 2001—at a time when Belgium did not allow either euthanasia or PAS. For the Netherlands, on the other hand (see Table 2.1), this rate stood at 0.7% in 1995 and had declined to 0.5% by 2005. As the authors of the study that collected these data conclude, "the fact that ending life without an explicit request is also practiced in countries where euthanasia is not legal suggests that other factors may be more important."[150]

Many foreign critics condemn the Netherlands for its practice of euthanasia, PAS, and other life-ending practices by contrasting the Dutch experience with an ideal situation in which this kind of medical behavior allegedly does not occur. In fact, abundant evidence shows that physicians' end-of-life decisions that result in the death of patients are widespread in all countries,[151] albeit largely hidden and, for the most part, without any kind of judicial scrutiny. The real difference is, that in the Netherlands, this behavior is carried out transparently, and that, at least as concerns euthanasia and PAS, is subject to some legal control. This system of control, like the enforcement of all laws everywhere, is imperfect. It also does not cover the large number of cases involving other end-of-life measures that, although often very similar to euthanasia, are categorized differently. Reliance on self-reporting assumes that most physicians do adhere to the prevailing standards of professional integrity. Yet, surely, an imperfect system of supervision is better than no legal control at all. This unfortunately is the situation in most other countries, where these life-shortening practices take place surreptitiously in an illegal and secret underground environment and therefore, for the most part, remain beyond the reach of the law.

Legal control over euthanasia and other end-of-life decisions in the Netherlands is not perfect, conclude Griffiths and his co-authors in their massive 2008 study of euthanasia in Europe . "However it is better than in other countries for which information is available, and it has been getting more encompassing, more refined, and in practice more effective in the two decades since euthanasia became legal." Legal changes have occurred, "almost all of it in the direction of clarifying and tightening the require-ments of due care and improving the system of control."[152]

Raphael Cohen-Amalgor, an Israeli observer of the Dutch scene, has spoken of a culture that "has a chilling effect on the open, critical debate."[153] Other scholars working in the field disagree with this find-ing.[154] John Griffiths and colleagues, writing in 1998, criticized their Dutch countrymen for often ignoring foreign criticism, although they saw rea-sons for this dismissive attitude. All too often, they write, the charges from abroad "have not been made in a way which invites serious response. Imprecision, exaggeration, suggestion and innuendo, misinterpretation and misrepresentation, ideological *ipse dixitism*, and outright lying and slander (not to speak of bad manners) have taken the place of careful analysis of the problem and consideration of Dutch evidence."[155]

Whatever the merits of this indictment, it certainly would appear that many foreign critics lack sufficient understanding and empathy for what the American scholar David Thomasma appropriately has called "the Euthanasia experience as it is lived."[156] In his book, subtitled "Inside the Dutch Debate About Euthanasia," he has provided telling accounts of how Dutch doctors themselves feel about the life-ending practices they are engaged in.

Unlike American doctor Jack Kevorkian, often with justice called a "traveling executioner," in these accounts, Dutch doctors come across as sensitive human beings from whom the practice of euthanasia and PAS often takes a heavy emotional toll. "Although I am grateful I am able to perform euthanasia for my patients," relates one doctor, "it is very diffi-cult for me. I believe euthanasia is part of my professional responsibility, but I am never comfortable with it. I have euthanized a half dozen patients, but it hurts each time because you cannot escape from the fact that you are taking a life." Several other doctors stated similarly that "con-trary to uninformed speculation," the act does not become easier over time. "Each of the euthanasias I have performed has been as different and difficult as if it were the first." Or, as another physician put it: "From experience, I can say it never gets any easier."[157]

Several doctors expressed their satisfaction with being able to help their suffering terminal patients in their hour of need. "I see euthanasia as part of the role of the physician. The duty of a doctor is to help patients come into the world, and comfort them. But also to help patients to exit the world as comfortably as possible. The duty of the doctor does not end even if there are no further treatment options to be offered. I see euthanasia as one of the ways I can care for my patients. For me, performing euthanasia is always based on the determination that this is the best I can do for my patient in the circumstances that prevail at the time. I see it as an overall benefit, not a harm." An oncologist noted that "even though the number of patients who choose it is very small, knowing that euthanasia is an option is a comfort for patients. It gives them power over the circumstances of their dying." In the words of another doctor: "Even if the time for euthanasia never comes, just the fact that the physician talks about it with the patient provides an assurance that makes dying a little easier. Patients know they will not be left alone in pain, they will not have to suffer unnecessarily, and they have the comfort of knowing their physician will be there for them no matter what."[158]

A Catholic doctor agreed that under some conditions "euthanasia is justified because it is the better of two terrible alternatives. Killing is always bad but it is not always the worst alternative. Patients find themselves in such terrible situations that a choice must be made between a bad action, killing, or a worse action, allowing the suffering to continue." Even though this doctor recognized that killing in some extreme circumstances is the better choice, he stated that he could not bring himself to do it. He had spent his entire professional career devoted to the preservation of life and to "waiver from that commitment now and take a life would be, I think, a violation of a deep-seated personal and professional credo. This commitment to life does not prevent me, in very extreme circumstances, from helping to arrange for my patient's euthanasia. The actual performance of the act I cannot do."[159]

According to available data, these anecdotal accounts are representative of the Dutch medical profession. A study of the emotional impact on physicians of hastening the death of a patient, published in 2001, revealed that 75% of doctors had a feeling of "discomfort" after their most recent case of euthanasia, and 58% expressed that same feeling after having assisted in the suicide of a patient. Of the 110 physicians who had performed euthanasia, 45% reported that their most recent case had been as difficult as the previous cases. At the same time, 95% of these doctors indicated their willingness to assist in the death of other patients in the future. The authors of the study concluded that the data collected "do not indicate that repeated performance [of euthanasia or PAS] 'numbs' the emotions or that this emotionally laden type of medical decision-making becomes part of 'normal' medical practice."[160] To assist in the death of a patient with due care is part of normal medical practice in the legal sense, but this does not mean that doctors consider these procedures as an unburdensome "normal" part of their medical calling, which is to cure disease and not to take lives.

The Dutch trust their doctors to stand by them in their hour of dire need. As the Dutch scholar G.A.M. Widdershoven puts it, "trust not only means that one can be sure that the physician will not misuse his or her power. It means first and foremost that one can be sure one will not be left alone in a hopeless situation. Concerning end-of-life issues, fear of abandonment is more pervasive in the Netherlands than fear of unwanted interventions by the physician. Patients express the need to be cared for, and not to be left alone to die. The values of support, trust and care," he concludes, "are central to Dutch euthanasia practice."[161]

The embrace of these values by the Dutch people, I would add, is in large measure the result of the long-term close relationship of family doctor and patient that exists in the Netherlands. Such close personal rapport between doctor and patient certainly does not prevail in the United States, where the medical profession has largely abandoned house calls and home care. This state of affairs could lead American physicians to adopt a far more perfunctory and less conscientious approach to euthanasia and PAS. If we add to that the high cost of medical care and the large number of uninsured or underinsured, which raises the danger that financial considerations will enter into the decision-making process in end-of-life care, we must conclude that the Dutch way of handling end-of-life issues is probably not easily transferable to countries like the United States. Whether the achievement of transparency by getting these practices out into the open and creating some oversight, control and accountability could outbalance these hazards of the legalization of euthanasia and/or PAS in the United States is a question to which I will return in a later chapter.

3

VOLUNTARY EUTHANASIA IN BELGIUM

On May 16, 2002, the Belgian House of Representatives, following the example of the Senate, approved a bill legalizing euthanasia. After the king had signed the legislation on May 28, it was published in the *Belgish Staatsblad* (the official Belgian gazette) on June 22, and became effective three months later on September 22, 2002. In contrast to the Netherlands, where a series of court cases over many years had made euthanasia and physician-assisted suicide (PAS) practices that carried little risk of prosecution and where both the medical profession and the public had come to accept these modes of assisted death, the adoption of the Belgian law was preceded by much acrimonious debate. As we will see, until 1999, no legislative majority for the legalization of euthanasia could be found. The process, once started, was short and characterized by strong polarization. Neither the courts nor the organized medical community had any part in the development of the legal norms that, within a short time, became the law on euthanasia.

How Belgium Legalized Euthanasia

In 1980, two right-to-die organizations were founded, one for each of the two language groups of the country. During the 1980s, public discussion of euthanasia gradually became acceptable, and several bills for the legalization of euthanasia were introduced by individual members of parliament. However, none of these bills received serious consideration, because, until the 1990s, the Christian Democratic parties, who dominated the government during the 1980s, rejected or blocked all attempts to regulate euthanasia.[1]

This does not mean that euthanasia was not practiced in Belgium during those years. We have no data on the frequency of end-of-life decisions for the whole of the country for that period, but available data for Flanders, the Dutch-speaking part of Belgium, where about 60% of the population lives, show that, before 2002, practices that aimed at ending the patient's life were frequent, including euthanasia and PAS, which were illegal. A survey of end-of-life decisions by physicians in Flanders between January 1 and April 30, 1998 showed that 0.2% of all deaths were the result of PAS and 1.1% the consequence of euthanasia. An additional 5.3% of all deaths involved the withholding or withdrawing of life-prolonging treatment with the explicit intention of shortening the patient's life. Most striking was the finding that in 3.1% of the cases the terminating of life had taken place without the patient's explicit request (LAWER or life-terminating act without explicit request). The figure of 3.1 % for LAWER was about four times as high as in the Netherlands, where at no time has it exceeded 0.8% of all deaths.[2] These results, wrote two students of the subject, "directly challenge the effectiveness of a policy of criminal prohibition in controlling euthanasia."[3]

There are several reasons for the high rate of LAWER during those years. A substantial number of physicians stated that consulting the patient would have done more harm than good and that proceeding to end life without explicit request was best for the patient. Data from a smaller study show that doctors with more than 20 years of experience chose to forego consulting their competent patients three times as often as did less-experienced doctors, seeming to indicate the presence of strong paternalistic sentiments on the part of older physicians in particular.[4] One of the authors of this study, Johan Bilsen, further surmises that fear of legal complications at a time when PAS and euthanasia were illegal probably made doctors proceed in a less than open manner and contributed to the high rate of LAWER.[5] The members of this research group expressed the same view in another publication: "Perhaps less attention is given to requirements of careful end-of-life practice in a society with a restrictive approach than in one with an open approach that tolerates and regulates euthanasia and PAS."[6] When the study of end-of-life decisions in

Flanders was repeated in 2001, it turned out that the rate of LAWER was less than half (1.5%) of what it had been in 1998. The greater attention to careful practice may have been related to the intensive debate preceding the legalization of euthanasia in 2002, and to the expectation that legalization was imminent. Such circumstances made it less necessary to act in a clandestine manner.[7]

Not only was the patient's participation in these crucial life-or-death decisions poorly respected during the years preceding legalization, but other practices similarly revealed a frequent violation of the requirements of careful and prudent practice. The majority of cases of euthanasia and PAS occurred in patients' homes. However, in more than half the cases where euthanasia took place in an institution, nurses administered the lethal medication, and in only 14% of these cases was a physician present while the nurse administered the drug. Nurses were involved in giving the lethal injection in 83% of the cases of LAWER in institutions, and in 43% of these cases the physician was absent. It is not clear whether the nurses administering these drugs at the request of physicians were always aware of the lethality of their act. Be that as it may, Johan Bilsen, who reports these occurrences, concludes that it is not "consistent with physicians' professional norms to delegate heavily consequential acts of this kind and, even more alarmingly, to do so without being present during or after the procedure."[8]

And there was more. The study of end-of-life practices in 1998 revealed that pharmacological practices varied widely. Eleven different products were used, with a wide range in doses and modes of administration. The time between administration of the lethal dose and the onset of death ranged from 4 minutes to 15 hours, and only in a small minority of cases were effective euthanatics used. Bilsen writes: "Most physicians, clandestinely engaging in euthanasia in Belgium, seemed unaware of procedures for guaranteeing a quick, mild, and certain death. . . . Our results indicate an inconsistent, poorly documented, and substandard medical approach to euthanasia in Flanders, Belgium in 1998."[9] Most of the deaths involving euthanasia or PAS were reported in the death certificates as deaths from natural causes.[10]

Support for the idea of bringing the euthanasia issue into the open gradually improved during the 1980s, because of a weakening of traditional values and a greater desire to find compassionate solutions to the long and arduous deaths that many terminal patients had to endure as a result of advances in medical technology. Although a substantial segment of the medical profession continued to oppose the legal control of euthanasia, public opinion began to shift in the direction of decriminalization. Data from the European Values Survey show that, between 1981 and 1999, support for euthanasia in Belgium increased by 69.1%, the largest increase in any European country and three times the average increase for all of Europe.[11]

In 1987, a colloquium, "Bioethics in the 1990s," was convened by the Minister for Health and the Handicapped, one of a growing number of Christian Democrats who had begun to adopt a more flexible position on end-of-life issues. During the closing days of this colloquium, the minister proposed the formation of an advisory committee on bioethics. It took several more years before this committee received the official go-ahead, but in 1996 the committee finally began its work.

The Belgian Advisory Committee on Bioethics (BBAB) was composed of 35 members from various disciplines—doctors, jurists, ethicists, psychologists, and sociologists. As is customary in Belgium, it was also representative of the two language groups in the country and of different ideological positions (i.e., it included an equal number of Catholics and nonreligious people). The mandate of the committee was to provide advice and information to society and the state on problems that arise as a result of medical advances and their implementation in the fields of biology, medicine, and health care, and to explore the ethical, social, and legal aspects of the issues involved.[12]

In May 1997, the BBAB issued its first set of recommendations, "Recommendation No. 1 of 12 May 1997 Concerning the Desirability of a Legal Recognition of Euthanasia." The Committee, adopting a Dutch formula of 1985, defined euthanasia as "intentionally terminating another person's life at that person's request." This was in line with the request of the presidents of the Senate and House of Representatives, who had asked for an opinion "on the desirability of a legal recognition of the termination of life at the request of the terminally ill patient (euthanasia)." The committee made it clear that its recommendations would be limited to euthanasia for competent terminal patients and carried out by a physician.[13]

True to its mandate to represent the different opinions within the committee, the BBAB proposed four possible ways of handling the issue of voluntary euthanasia:

1. Euthanasia carried out by a physician using appropriate safeguards of due care to protect patients would be decriminalized.
2. Euthanasia would remain unlawful but physicians could claim a "situation of necessity," similar to the way in which courts in the Netherlands had come to deal with cases of euthanasia during the 1980s and 1990s.
3. Laws would regulate all end-of-life decisions, with euthanasia again being allowed under the claim of necessity.
4. The present prohibition of euthanasia would be upheld.

The recommendations of the BBAB were discussed in the Senate in December 1997, but action on a concrete legislative proposal was postponed pending the receipt of advice regarding incompetent patients. This report, "Recommendation No. 9 Concerning Termination of Life of Incompetent Patients," was finally issued in February 1999 and revealed a sharply split committee. Some members favored the legal recognition of euthanasia for incompetent patients, with or without an advance directive requesting termination of life in situations of incompetence. Others wanted to limit euthanasia to patients who had an advance directive in place, while still others opposed any change in the current law that prohibited the termination of life for incompetent patients.[14]

The resulting deadlock was broken with the election of June 1999, in which the Christian Democratic parties that had dominated Belgian politics for several decades suffered a stunning defeat. The new government, formed by the Liberals, Socialists, and Greens (the so-called the "purplegreen" or "rainbow" coalition), quickly made it clear that it was prepared to act decisively on the issue of euthanasia. There followed the introduction of several bills in the Senate that, by December 1999, were consolidated into a joint bill sponsored by the majority parties. Between February and May 2000, hearings were held before the Joint Committee for Justice and Social Affairs, followed by a sharply polarized debate in the committee that lasted until March 2001. During this debate, the Christian Democrats proposed several hundred amendments, most of which were rejected by the majority parties in control of the proceedings. On March 20, 2001, finally, the Joint Committee by a vote of 17 to 12 approved a euthanasia bill. Although strongly supported by the Catholic organization Caritas Flanders, which coordinates the work of Catholic hospitals in Flanders, and the Flemish Palliative Care Federation, the draft bill did not include the requirement of a prior palliative consultation (a "palliative filter"). However, a separate bill stressing the importance of palliative care was adopted unanimously.[15]

The chairman of the Senate, concerned about the moral implications of the euthanasia bill, forwarded the legislation to the Council of State, an advisory body for pending legislation, but the council declined to hold up the bill. During debate by the full Senate, 136 more amendments were offered, most of them by the opposition Christian Democrats, but none was approved. The final vote, which came on October 25, 2001, reflected the existing polarization. Forty-four votes were in favor of the legalization of euthanasia, with two abstentions, and 22 votes against—all dissenting votes from senators belonging to the opposition. The vote was equally divided in the House of Representatives. Here, too, none of the about 100 amendments that had been proposed during the preceding debate was approved. When the lower chamber voted on May 16, 2002, there were 86 votes for the bill, 10 abstentions, and 51 votes against the legalization of euthanasia. A last attempt to kill the legislation was made by two pro-life organizations that, in December 2002, took the law on euthanasia to the Court of Arbitration (since 2007 called the Constitutional Court), but this court rejected their petition in an opinion consisting of three paragraphs issued on January 14, 2004.[16]

The Law on Euthanasia of May 28, 2002

The Belgian euthanasia law[17] defines euthanasia "as intentionally terminating life by someone other than the person concerned, at the latter's request" (Section 2). The "someone" must be a physician, as becomes clear in Section 3, which states that a physician who performs euthanasia commits no criminal offence when he or she ensures that

- the patient has attained the age of majority and is legally competent and conscious at the moment of making the request;

- the request is voluntary, well-considered, and repeated, and is not the result of any external pressure;
- the patient is in a medically futile condition of constant and unbearable physical or mental suffering that can not be alleviated, resulting from a serious and incurable disorder caused by illness or accident.

Before carrying out the act of euthanasia, the physician must also

- Explain to the patient his or her medical condition and life expectancy, and discuss options other than euthanasia, such as palliative care. Both patient and doctor must conclude that no alternatives to euthanasia are available and that the patient's request is completely voluntary.
- Be certain of the patient's physical or mental suffering and of the durable nature of the request for euthanasia. To this end, the physician must have several conversations with the patient, spread over a reasonable period of time.
- Consult another doctor, not connected to the patient or the attending physician and competent to give an opinion about the disease in question, who must review the patient's record and examine the patient. This independent physician must likewise conclude that the patient's suffering, physical or mental, is constant and unbearable and cannot be alleviated.
- Discuss the request of the patient with any nursing team that has regular contact with the patient.
- Discuss the request with any relatives chosen by the patient.
- Be certain that the patient has had the opportunity to discuss his or her request with any person he or she chooses.

If the physician believes that the patient is not expected to die in the near future (is not in a terminal stage of the illness), he or she must also

- Consult a second physician who is a specialist in the disorder in question. This doctor, after examining the patient, must likewise be convinced that the conditions enumerated above have been satisfied.
- Must allow at least one month between the patient's request and the act of euthanasia.

The patient's request for euthanasia must be in written form. If the patient is incapable of writing, the document can be drawn up by a person who has no material interest in the death of the patient. The patient can revoke this request at any time (Section 3).

The law allows a person to draw up a written advance directive that will authorize a physician to carry out the act of euthanasia if, in the future, the patient suffers from a serious and incurable disorder, becomes unconscious, and this condition is irreversible. Such a directive also constitutes a power of attorney for designated persons to inform the physician of the patient's wishes. The advance directive must be drafted or reconfirmed no more than five years prior to the person's loss of ability to express his or her wishes. The physician must adhere to all the conditions and procedures enumerated in the law, although, since such patients are not assumed capable of suffering, the requirement of unbearable suffering is waived (Section 4).

For the implementation of the law, a Federal Control and Evaluation Commission is established, consisting of 16 members, appointed by the council of ministers for a term of four years. Eight of these commissioners are to be doctors of medicine, four professors of law or practicing lawyers, and four are to be drawn from groups that deal with the problems of incurable patients. Each linguistic group is to have at least three candidates of each sex.

The Commission is to draft a registration form, which is to be submitted to the Commission by a physician performing euthanasia within four working days. The first part of this form must include the names and addresses of the patient, of the attending physician, and of the physician and others consulted. The second part includes demographic data of the patient, details about his condition and the act of euthanasia, as well as assurances that the conditions and procedures required by the law have been fulfilled. The first part of the document is to be put into a sealed envelope, and will be opened only if a majority of the Commission decides that the act of euthanasia was carried out without compliance with the conditions of prudent practice stipulated in the law. In that case, the Commission can either request additional information from the attending physician, or, if approved by a two-thirds majority, hand the case over to the public prosecutor of the jurisdiction where the patient died (Sections 5–8).

Every two years, the Commission is also required to submit a report to parliament containing statistical information about the cases handled and any suggestions for changes in the law (Section 9). The law contains a conscience clause—no physician may be compelled to perform euthanasia, and no other person may be compelled to assist in the performance of euthanasia (Section 14). Subsequent rulings by the Control Commission have made it clear that the law does not apply to normal medical practice, such as foregoing further treatment or pain relief that results in a shortening of life. On the other hand, the administration of narcotics at elevated levels constitutes euthanasia if the patient has requested it.[18]

The Belgian law on euthanasia undoubted owes much to Dutch practice and legislation, but there are also some important differences. The Belgian act covers both somatic and psychiatric diseases, the patient must be over 18 years old (although the National Disciplinary Board of the Order of Physicians, authorized to promulgate rules of conduct for the medical profession, is said to have mitigated this requirement[19]), the advance directive cannot be older than five years or must be reconfirmed after five years, and the law explicitly states that the unbearable suffering must be due to "illness or accident," thus ruling out cases of existential suffering as in the Dutch *Brongersma* case of 1998.

Perhaps the most striking difference between the Belgian and Dutch law is the omission of PAS from the Belgian legislation. John Griffiths and colleagues surmise that this happened because, during the debate preceding adoption, opponents of the law regarded PAS as simply killing somebody on demand, and supporters, who had a tough fight as it was, did not want to be seen as supporting something so "frivolous."[20] Whatever the reasons for the omission, in March 2003, the Order of Physicians decided that PAS was equivalent to euthanasia as long as the conditions and procedures of the Law on euthanasia were adhered to, and in 2004, the Control Commission agreed with this view. The law of 2002, the Commission declared, did not specify the practicalities of euthanasia.[21] This assessment, note Griffiths and colleagues appropriately, is not entirely sound, for the law is about euthanasia, defined as "terminating life by *someone other than the person* [italics added] concerned."[22] There is also Par. 422 of the Criminal Code, which makes it a crime not to help a person in danger.

This clause could be invoked against a physician who not only fails to prevent a danger such as suicide but actually facilitates it.[23] However, the Commission probably has the last word in these matters.

As mentioned earlier, in addition to the law on euthanasia, parliament also was presented with a law on palliative care. This legislation, approved on June 14, 2002, did not include the "palliative filter" for euthanasia sought by Caritas Flanders and others, but it did state that "all patients are entitled to benefit from palliative care at the end of their life." The attending physician is obligated to inform the patient of the availability of such care, including physical, psychological, social, and moral support that will optimize the quality of life during the time the patient has left (Section 2).[24] Even though the law was formulated in general terms, it did constitute a formal recognition of the importance of palliative care, and this endorsement undoubtedly has helped advance palliative care in the country. I will return to this subject later in this chapter. At the same time, it should be noted, palliative care is not a substitute for euthanasia. The patient, as the federal control commission has ruled, has the right to refuse treatment, and this includes palliative care.[25]

The Federal Control Commission is empowered to suggest changes in the euthanasia law, but so far there has been only one formal amendment. On November 10, 2005, a new article 3bis was added providing greater legal security for pharmacists who supply the legal medication. Doctors are required to state in writing that they have fulfilled all conditions of the law, and pharmacists enjoy legal immunity even if the physician later is charged in an illegal death.[26]

The Practice of Euthanasia Since 2002

Unlike the situation in the Netherlands, as of this writing, we have relatively few empirical studies of how the Belgian system of euthanasia is working. Some useful information can be found in the three biannual reports of the Federal Control Commission, issued in 2004, 2006, and 2008.[27] The data in Tables 3.1–3.3 are based on this source.

During the six years covered, the number of cases reported to the Commission has increased, which is considered a result of the fact that the law gradually has become better known (Table 3.1).

TABLE 3.1 Cases of Euthanasia

	2002*–2003	2004–2005	2006–2007
Total number of reported cases	259	742	924
Euthanasia as percentage of all deaths	0.2%	0.36%	0.44%
Flemish-/Dutch-speaking	83%	86%	81%
French-speaking	17%	14%	19%

*Since the law went into effect on September 22, 2002, data for the year 2002 include only the period from September 22, 2002 to December 31, 2003.

TABLE 3.2 Characteristics of Patients Choosing Euthanasia

	2002*–2003	2004–2005	2006–2007
Sex:			
Male	50%	54%	54%
Female	50	46	46
Age (number of cases):			
Below 20	1	2	1
20–39	8	45	24
40–59	83	209	231
60–79	125 (48%)	362 (49%)	505 (55%)
80 and above	42	124	163
Life Expectancy:			
Brief	92%	93%	94%
Not-brief (more than 1 month)	8	7	6
Diagnosis:			
Cancer	83%	83%	81%
Neuromuscular diseases	12	6	8
Other	5	11	11

*Since the law went into effect on September 22, 2002, data for the year 2002 include only the period from September 22, 2002 to December 31, 2003.

TABLE 3.3 Decisions of the Control Commission

	2002*–2003	2004–2005	2006–2007
Report accepted	69%	78%	80%
Remarks sent to physician	12	5	7
Additional information requested	19	17	13
Sent to public prosecutor	0	0	0

*Since the law went into effect on September 22, 2002, data for the year 2002 include only the period from September 22, 2002 to December 31, 2003.

Although the number of cases of euthanasia has increased over the years, according to these figures, euthanasia takes place in Belgium far less frequently than in the Netherlands, where it has never been less than 1.7% of all deaths. In Belgium, practically all reported cases of euthanasia took place as a result of a direct personal request, rather than on the basis of an advance directive by an unconscious patient: 99.5% in 2002–2004, 98% in 2004–2005, and 96% in 2006–2007. Given the legal ambiguity of PAS in the Belgian law, it is not surprising that the number of reported cases of PAS is no more than 1% of all cases of assisted death.[28]

Table 3.1 shows that the great majority of reported cases of euthanasia have come from the Dutch-speaking part of Belgium. Even though 60% of the Belgian population is Dutch-speaking, these figures show a considerable disparity. According to commissioner Marc Englert, it is difficult to find a conclusive reason for this difference. Among the possible explanations is the fact that physicians in the French-speaking part of Belgium carried out fewer acts of euthanasia for cancer patients. Another factor may be different attitudes toward death in the two language regions of the country.[29] On the basis of research in both parts of the country, Lieve Van den Block has noted that in the Dutch-speaking community, "physicians, patients or their families seem to be more readily prepared to make or ask for life-shortening decisions than in the French-speaking community."[30] Still another reason explaining the difference between the two populations may be the fact that "French-speaking physicians, especially general practitioners, seem to report their cases less often to the Federal Evaluation and Control Commission than the Dutch-speaking."[31] (Since about 75% of Belgians in both language regions are Roman Catholic, religion does not appear to be a factor in explaining this difference.)

Contrary to the fears of some feminists and organizations of senior citizens, women and the very old have not been over-represented, and other characteristics of the persons choosing euthanasia similarly reveal nothing of note.

About half of all reported cases of euthanasia took place in hospitals, and a somewhat smaller number in homes. None of the cases of euthanasia reported to the Commission showed imprudent practice (i.e., a violation of the conditions and procedures required by the law), although in a substantial number of cases the Commission, after opening the envelope containing the identity of the doctor, contacted the physician either with remarks or with a request for additional information (see Table 3.3). The scrutiny of the Commission thus is clearly not merely a formality.

Nothing is known of the nature of the remarks sent to physicians or of the kind of additional information requested by the Commission. Unlike in the Netherlands, therefore, the reports of the Commission do not provide feedback to the medical profession that could improve the quality of the euthanasia practice nor do they afford a basis for informed public assessment of the functioning of the Commission. In short, the Griffiths team concludes, "a commission whose raison d'être is to produce transparency and thereby maintain confidence in euthanasia practice, itself suffers from a regrettable absence of transparency."[32]

The Control Commission depends on the voluntary cooperation of doctors, but unfortunately we have no data that would enable us to establish to what extent the *reported* cases coincide with the *actual* number of cases euthanasia and PAS. The Griffiths team used the number of cases that occurred in Flanders in 1998 and compared that figure with the number of cases reported in 2005. Assuming that the frequency of euthanasia had remained constant, they arrived at a reporting rate of 47%.[33] According to the European End-of-Life (EURELD) study, 0.31% of all deaths in Belgium (Flanders) between June 2001 and February 2002 were the result of euthanasia and PAS.[34] Reports received by the Control Commission, on the other hand, indicate that, between September 22, 2002 and December 31, 2003, cases of euthanasia (with 83% of these reports coming from Flanders) represented 0.2% of all deaths. These figures would yield a reporting rate of 65%. Standing against these low reporting figures (ranging from 47% to 65%), we have the third report of the Control Commission, published in 2008, which stated that in their view the number of clandestine cases of euthanasia was small.[35] In the absence of relevant data, there exists no way to reconcile these findings.

Unlike in the Netherlands, where the practice of euthanasia enjoys strong support from the medical profession, such broad support does not exist in Belgium. Data from the EURELD survey, collected in the second half of 2002, show that only 6.1% of Roman Catholic doctors had ever performed PAS or euthanasia, and even among nonreligious doctors the rate was no higher than 25.6%.[36] The fact that Belgian doctors have strong reservations about euthanasia may have a negative influence on the rate at which physicians report cases of euthanasia. From the point of view of many physicians, the euthanasia law was imposed on the medical profession and exemplifies the intrusion of politics into the practice of medicine. Before the enactment of the euthanasia law, the Order of Physicians, established by law to regulate the medical profession and responsible for professional discipline, had rejected euthanasia. Article 95 of the Code of Medical Deontology prohibited doctors from providing any assistance in dying.[37]

After the legalization of euthanasia, the Order of Physicians grudgingly accepted the new situation. In a statement issued in March 2003, the National Council of the Order of Physicians noted: "When in a democratic state a law [on ethical issues] is established and this law respects the freedom of conscience of each physician, the existence of this law cannot be ignored by a public institution such as the Order of Physicians." Three years later, finally, the Order of Physicians modified Article 95 of the Code of Medical Deontology. In a somewhat ambiguous manner, the revised Articles 95–98 now state that when receiving a question regarding the end of life, a physician should mention all possible options and provide any medical and moral assistance required.[38]

The Association of General Practitioners has taken a clearer and more positive position. According to a "Policy Statement on End of Life Decisions and Euthanasia," issued together with the Academic Center for General Practice/Family Medicine at the Catholic University of Leuven and the Academy for Knowledge at the University of Ghent on December 4, 2003, "the responsibilities of the general practitioner include aid in dying and everything connected thereto." One of the possible choices of dying is euthanasia, which should be included in the total palliative care made available to a patient. The statement rejected the creation of special "euthanasia teams and centres" and instead proposed the formation of interdisciplinary palliative teams that include psychological and/or spiritual care in a unified palliative care program for dying patients. In sum, the Association of General Practitioners, in agreement with the Flemish Federation for Palliative Care, regards euthanasia and palliative care not as opposites and instead sees euthanasia to be part of palliative care, which the attending doctor and a multidisciplinary care team organize at the end of a patient's life.[39]

In 2003, a consultation program very similar to the Dutch Support and Consultation in the Netherlands (SCEN) program was set up in the Flemish part of Belgium. It is known as Forum for End-of-Life Information (LEIF) and includes about 200 physicians with special training in end-of-life care, including palliative care and euthanasia. In 2006, a similar program was set up for nurses, and in 2007, an organization equivalent to LEIF, Médecins EOL, was established in Wallonia, the French-speaking segment of Belgium. So far, no information is available on the impact of these advisory teams on the practice of euthanasia.[40]

A prior palliative consultation as a condition of euthanasia is the main defining feature of the position of the Catholic organization Caritas Flanders, an umbrella organization founded in 1932 for 62 general hospitals, 94 mental health care institutions, 326 geriatric care institutions, 397 facilities for handicapped persons, and 344 facilities for public welfare. These institutions represent about 65% of general hospitals and 40% of nursing homes, and serve a population of about 6 million people. While the euthanasia legislation was still in the drafting stage, the ethics committee of Caritas, made up of physicians, nurses, directors of health care institutions, ethicists, jurists, and pastoral workers, began preparing a set of guidelines for clinical practice. A draft, prepared by the secretary of the committee, Professor Chris Gastmans of the Center for Biomedical Ethics and Law at the Catholic University of Leuven, was widely circulated, and these discussions included the Flemish Palliative Care Federation. As a result of these deliberations, the concept of the "palliative filter" was developed. The draft guidelines were presented to the Board of Directors of Caritas Flanders, and were approved on April 26, 2002.[41]

As mentioned earlier, the requirement of a palliative filter, urged by Caritas Flanders but opposed by the right-to-die organizations, did not make it into the euthanasia law. Immediately following the approval of the legislation, the guidelines were sent to the 1,213 Caritas-affiliated institutions, and they now govern the practice of practically all of these institutions.[42] According to the guidelines, the competent, terminally ill person who suffers severely and requests euthanasia should be provided with the expertise of a specialized palliative support team. This team should address the medical, as well as the mental and spiritual well-being of the patient. If the pain and distress of the terminal patient cannot be controlled by the use of normal palliative methods, and the patient's suffering is enormous and prevents a dignified death, palliative sedation should be considered. Palliative sedation in this context involves the intentional administration of sedative drugs in dosages required to reduce the consciousness of a terminal patient as much as necessary in order to relieve his refractory symptoms.

The request of a patient for euthanasia must lead to a searching examination of all aspects of the patient's situation—his diagnosis and prognosis, mental competence, the reaction of family and friends—but it is to be treated seriously. On the other hand, the patient's request in and by itself is a necessary but not a sufficient reason for initiating euthanasia. The attending physician must ensure that all existing possibilities for palliative care are explored, and must discuss the euthanasia request with the institution's palliative support team and the nursing team. If the patient persists in his request for euthanasia despite the implementation of this palliative filter procedure, the attending physician will relieve the patient's suffering by preparing for euthanasia. He or she must adhere to the legal criteria of Section 3 of the euthanasia law, including a consultation with second physician.[43]

The position on euthanasia taken by Caritas, it should be noted, is in conflict with the declaration of the Belgian Roman Catholic bishops issued on May 16, 2002, which flatly rejected the acceptability of euthanasia under any circumstances.[44] In defense of Caritas' qualified acceptance of euthanasia, Chris Gastmans and his co-authors have stressed the importance of developing a conception of human dignity "that is accessible for nonbelievers and at the same time expresses the basic moral intuitions of every Christian." Moreover, they stressed, although the teaching of the Roman Catholic Magisterium contains values and principles that hold *in general* for a problem such as euthanasia, *concrete cases* create exceptional circumstances. For that reason, they concluded, the Magisterium's pronouncements on ethics "are almost never normatively binding" in these exceptional circumstances. Christian health care institutions must anchor their ethics in "clinical caring practices on the one hand and the Christian story on the other. The starting point is that Christian ethics implies 'ever greater human dignity.'" By requiring a palliative filter as a prior condition of euthanasia, they pointed out, Caritas Flanders has been able to provide adequate protection to the human person while at the same time reducing the number of persistent requests for euthanasia to a strict minimum.[45]

The Belgian law allows euthanasia not only for physical but also for "mental suffering," but Catholic institutions reject euthanasia in such cases. In fact, because of the requirement that a request for euthanasia be "voluntary, well-considered, and repeated" the number of requests from psychiatric patients is reported to be small.[46] Unlike in the Netherlands, Belgian professional organizations have not provided guidelines on how to handle such cases. When, on March 19, 2008, Hugo Maurice Julien Claus, one of the most important contemporary Flemish authors and in the very early stage of Alzheimer's disease, died as a result of euthanasia, the issue of assisted death for patients with various kinds of dementia became the subject of wide public discussion. The Flemish Minister of Culture expressed understanding for Claus' desire to depart with "pride and dignity," whereas the Belgian Alzheimer League and Cardinal Godfried Danneels voiced criticism.[47]

The authors of the Caritas guidelines have acknowledged the important contribution of the Flemish Palliative Care Federation (FPZV) to the development of the palliative filter idea. The FPZV shares the important assumption of the euthanasia law that there will always be persons who, on their deathbed, will be afflicted with sustained and intolerable pain and distress. However, the organization argues, the assumption that in this situation the only choice is between inhumane dying and euthanasia ignores the contribution of specialized multidisciplinary palliative care. Such care can preempt and prevent many requests for euthanasia.[48]

According to the FPZV, it is a mistake to assume that the average physician or hospital ward possesses the necessary expertise to provide state-of-the-art palliative care. In the absence of such expertise, an informed choice for euthanasia is impossible, and many requests for euthanasia are in fact camouflaging a lack of palliative care. Even in the matter of pain control for incurably ill patients, medical treatment often exhibits grave shortcomings. There are also people who are tired of seemingly endless medical procedures and prefer to opt out. "But everyday dealings with dying people has taught the caregivers of the FPZV that only a very small minority of patients requesting euthanasia belong to this category. With the vast majority of patients requesting euthanasia, the request vanishes after they have encountered the beneficial effects produced by good palliative care." Hence, to avoid those pseudo-choices for euthanasia that result from lack of adequate palliative care, it is necessary to introduce the palliative filter, a prior palliative consultation, as a condition of euthanasia.[49]

The relatively high level of specialized palliative care existing in Belgium, it has been suggested, makes the requirement of a palliative filter a realistic option.[50] By 1999, Belgium had the second largest per capita number of beds for palliative care in Europe (after the United Kingdom).[51] Following the passage of the law on palliative care (at the same time as the law on euthanasia), the budget for palliative care was doubled, and this has helped in the development of a comprehensive palliative care network. To organize palliative care, the country is divided into 30 regions, and in each region a palliative network or local palliative care cooperative is responsible for the coordination of palliative care and for developing specific initiatives. Linked to each network or cooperative are multidisciplinary support teams for palliative care in the home, for hospitals, and for nursing homes. Each region also has a small inpatient palliative care unit. The system employs 14 full-time and 879 part-time physicians as well 3,238 nurses engaged full- or part-time in palliative care.[52] By 2007, Belgium ranked third among 52 countries in palliative care resources (after Iceland and the United Kingdom).[53]

A survey of general practitioners conducted in 2005–2006 showed that 41% of all non–sudden death patients, 61% of all cancer death patients, and 21% of all patients dying from diseases other than cancer received specialist multidisciplinary palliative care in their last weeks of life—ratios that are considered high.[54] The experience of a palliative care unit in Brussels appears to support the effectiveness of palliative care in reducing the number of requests for euthanasia. Between September 22, 2002 and December 31, 2003, only 35 of 510 patients in the unit (7%) asked for euthanasia, and in only 16 cases (3.1%) did such a request result in euthanasia.[55]

On the other hand, the survey of general practitioners in 2005–2006 revealed that euthanasia and PAS were more prevalent in inpatient palliative care units than in hospitals or nursing homes, and receiving spiritual care (part of palliative care) was also associated with higher frequencies of euthanasia and PAS than was receiving little or no spiritual care. Interpreting these findings, Lieve Van den Block surmises that palliative care enhances patient autonomy and may help patients express their wishes, including requests for euthanasia, more freely. The availability of palliative care services, she concludes, does not seem to prevent life-shortening measures such as euthanasia. "End-of-life decisions and palliative care do not seem to contradict, but if anything seem to reinforce each other."[56]

Further research may clarify these issues. As mentioned earlier and in contrast to the Netherlands, we have relatively few empirical data on the practice of euthanasia in Belgium. Most of the data that we do have come from the Control Commission, and we do not know to what extent the cases reported to the Commission coincide with the actual cases of euthanasia. Several studies now under way will hopefully yield a more complete picture of how euthanasia is being implemented in Belgium.

4

ASSISTED SUICIDE IN SWITZERLAND

According to the Swiss criminal code, neither suicide nor assisted suicide is illegal, per se. Article 114 makes it a criminal offense to kill a person upon request (i.e., to engage in mercy killing or voluntary euthanasia). However, assisting a person to commit suicide, states Article 115, is punishable only if done "for selfish motives."[1] In other jurisdictions where assisted suicide is legal—the Netherlands, Belgium, and Oregon—only physicians are allowed to engage in this practice, and this requirement is considered an important safeguard. In Switzerland, on the other hand, actual assistance in suicide can be and usually is performed by nonphysicians.

For reasons that are not fully understood, Switzerland has a suicide rate higher than the European average. According to the European End-of-Life (EURELD) study, it also has the highest rate of various end-of-life decisions, such as foregoing or not starting treatment, as well as of physician-assisted suicide (PAS). The EURELD study revealed that 0.36% of all deaths were the result of PAS, as compared to the runner-up, the Netherlands, which had a rate of 0.21%.[2] To be sure, most cases of assisted death in the Netherlands involve euthanasia rather than PAS, but that does not explain why Switzerland had a higher rate of PAS than the other countries studied (Belgium, Denmark, Italy, and Sweden).

One important reason for the high Swiss rate of PAS is the presence of several right-to-die organizations that offer this service. According to data collected by the Swiss federal government, during 2003, the three largest of these organizations facilitated PAS for 272 Swiss residents and 91 foreigners, for a total of 362 cases.[3] By contrast, there were 341 cases of PAS in the state of Oregon during ten years under the 1997 Death with Dignity Act.

Exit—German Switzerland: Association for a Humane Death

The largest Swiss right-to-die organization, Exit—German Switzerland, was founded in 1982, by Hedwig Zürcher, a retired teacher in Canton Zurich. Both the purpose and name of the organization were inspired by the Voluntary Euthanasia Society, Exit, established in London by Arthur Koestler in 1935. At its beginning, Exit merely provided a suicide manual. On January 15, 1985, executive director Rolf Sigg and his wife for the first time also provided actual assistance in suicide to a member of Exit.[4] Since about 1990, the organization, a member of the World Federation of Right-to-Die Societies, makes such assistance available to its members on a regular basis. Today, Exit has more than 50,000 members.

The practice of providing actual assistance in suicide at times has caused considerable debate and dissension within Exit, especially over the role of doctors in deciding for or against a request for assisted suicide and with regard to the kinds of persons who should be assisted. Between 1984 and 1997, the office of executive director had been filled by Protestant minister Rolf Sigg. Together with Dr. Meinrad Schär, a professor of preventive medicine at Zurich University and for many years the president of Exit, both men strongly affirmed the autonomy and absolute right of self-determination of patients against what they considered the exorbitant power of physicians. Publicist Peter Holenstein, who succeeded Sigg as executive director in 1997, on the other hand, saw the need for more control. He wanted formal training by physicians and psychologists for *Sterbehelfer* or *Freitodbegleiter* (assistants in suicide), insisted on contacting the treating physician, and favored soliciting a second opinion before agreeing to assist in a suicide. This stance drew sharp denunciation from the old guard, and at the annual meeting in May 1998, Holenstein was relieved of his office by a vote of 563 to 138.[5]

Although Sigg and Schär had prevailed over their critic, a large number of members criticized the dismissal of Holenstein as a threat to professionalism and transparency, and, disgusted with constant in-fighting, left the organization. One of these was human rights lawyer Ludwig A. Minelli, who, following his withdrawal from Exit, founded a new organization called Dignitas. During the following years, Exit managed to win new members, but the affair had caused damage. Ten years later, as we will see, a dispute over the same issues led to the resignation of well-known Swiss public figure Andreas Blum, who had served as official spokesman and director of Exit.

As another setback to Exit, in 1998, Dr. Schär was reprimanded by the Zurich Board of Health. In the case of a mentally ill patient in Basel, Schär was said to have prescribed a lethal medication based upon a questionable diagnosis. The Zurich authorities reminded the doctor that before prescribing medications patients had to be examined and a medical file established. Because Schär had failed to do so, he was deprived of his prescription rights until the completion of a criminal investigation of his conduct.[6]

The Basel case led to much public criticism of Exit. The president of Exit, Rudolf Syz, resigned over the incident because, as he stated, he could no longer head an organization in which such abuses took place. The Basel case, he feared, probably was not the only one of its kind. Syz also expressed his concern over the high sums of money Exit directors were drawing; he believed that working for Exit should be an honor, and he himself had never requested a single franc. Syz said that, for all these reasons, he no longer wanted to have anything to do with Exit.[7]

In 1999, the board of directors declared a moratorium (the so-called *Solothurner Erklärung)* on assisting patients with psychiatric problems. This decision was not well received by large numbers of Exit members who favored an easier, rather than a more circumscribed, access to assisted death. Many rank-and-file members to this day want to be able to acquire the lethal medication without a doctor's prescription.[8] Among those who criticized the moratorium was psychiatrist Peter Baumann, who left Exit in 2002 and founded his own rival organization, *Suizidhilfe* (Assistance with Suicide).

After a referendum of the membership of Exit showed that a majority of members regarded the moratorium as discriminatory, Exit solicited an expert assessment on the question of whether patients with mental disorders could be considered competent to request assistance in suicide. This expert opinion concluded that, although most psychiatric patients indeed sought suicide as a result of their mental illness, in some cases such patients could be considered competent.[9] In 2004, Exit thereupon loosened the moratorium and decided that requests for assisted suicide from psychiatric patients would not be automatically rejected.[10] The Federal Court of Justice (*Bundesgericht*), the highest court of appeal, relied upon the same expert assessment when, in 2006, it affirmed the legality of assisted death for competent psychiatric patients.[11] I will return to this issue later in this chapter.

This was not the end of unrest within the Exit organization. In 2001, Exit again saw a decline in membership as a result of charges that the directors had received excessively high compensation for their expenses.[12] The person in charge of the *Sterbehelfer*, Protestant minister Werner Kriesi, was said to draw a generous salary, whereas *Sterbehelfer* themselves were working as unpaid volunteers. Many of them were said to be demoralized and planned to quit.[13]

The qualifications of the assistants to suicide and the other issues raised by Holenstein also continued to occupy some members, and in the fall of 2007, these matters received wide publicity when highly regarded Exit board member Andreas Blum, a former director of Swiss Radio DRS, resigned his office in protest against what he regarded as consistent violation of Exit's principles and guidelines by the organization's leadership.

Blum announced his resignation from Exit's Board of Directors on October 15, 2007. When Exit president Hans Wehrli let it be known that Blum had resigned for reasons of "age," Blum went public, and in an interview with Michael Meier in the newspaper *Tagesanzeiger* termed Wehrli's statement "a lie," stating that he had resigned because he was no longer prepared to share the responsibility for certain dangerous developments in Exit. Among these was the elevation of human autonomy to the highest good, irrespective of legal order. The federal government, Blum argued, should assume the responsibility of regulating organizations like Exit to make sure that every assisted death involved competent individuals. He was disturbed by the continuing agitation for free access to lethal medication and the support for this clearly illegal practice by some Exit officials. The blind confidence in personal self-determination also manifested itself in the accumulation of reserve portions of the lethal medication natrium-pentobarbital (NaP), a violation of the regulations governing the dispensing of narcotics. Many of Exit's personnel considered themselves above the law.[14]

Matters had come to a head, Blum stated, when the president of Exit called Ludwig Minelli, the head of the assisted death organization Dignitas, an "idealist." Minelli, according to Blum, ran his outfit as a business and one-man show. It was unacceptable to leave decisions in life-and-death situations to the conscience of one person. Officials of Exit at times had referred foreigners (whom Exit does not accept) and others to Dignitas, and such a working relationship with an unscrupulous organization like Dignitas damaged Exit's own credibility and reputation.[15]

In a statement released on November 15, 2007, Exit's board of directors rejected Blum's criticism as unjustified, but Blum stood by his charges. In an interview with another newspaper a few days later, Blum insisted that Exit should extend its assistance only to fully competent individuals, whose suffering was truly unbearable, and whose wish to die was persistent and well-considered. In questions of doubt, the decision should always be in favor of rejecting the request. State regulation was needed to assure certain minimum standards for the performance of assisted death, financial transparency, and the adequate qualifications of assistants to suicide.[16]

How much merit is there in Blum's charges? How does Exit discharge its responsibility in these weighty life-and-death matters? We lack the information to answer these questions fully. According to a research team led by Georg Bosshard of the Institute of Legal Medicine at Zurich University, which was given access to all Exit records of assistance to suicide from 1990–2000, Exit files, especially those from the early years studied, contain little "specific data on the motivation, duration, and persistence of the wish to die, on the stage of disease and therapeutic options tried or offered, and the psychological setting."[17] Still, although the empirical record is incomplete, information is available from a variety of sources, including Exit publications, on a range of pertinent issues.

Membership in Exit is open to all Swiss citizens at least 18 years old, and to foreigners who reside in Switzerland. As a rule, applications for assistance in suicide from abroad are not accepted. According to Exit, the most important reasons for the adoption of this policy are that, in the case of foreign applicants it is not possible to achieve a clear picture of the reasons for the wish to die and because acceptance of foreigners would create the suspicion that the organization seeks financial gain from its work. Exit reserves the right to help those foreign citizens with close relations to Swiss members of the organization. The yearly membership fee is CHF 35 or CHF 600 for a lifetime membership.[18]

By the end of 2007, Exit had 52,695 members. Of these, 3,350 had joined in 2007.[19] The organization helps its members in two ways. First, it provides advance directives (also known as living wills), in which members state how they are to be treated by their doctors in case they are no longer able to articulate their wishes. Exit suggests that the directive be reconfirmed every two to three years and that the organization be empowered to enforce the directive if this should become necessary. The advance directive cannot be used to request assistance in suicide. Such assistance is available only to persons who ask for it directly. Second, Exit assists in suicide if three conditions are present: the person is competent, the desire to die is stated persistently, and the suffering is unbearable.[20] Even though Exit does not consider the latter activity—assisted suicide—as its most important, it is of course this feature that gives the organization its special character. Advance directives are noncontroversial and are available from many other sources.

A study of Exit cases in Canton Zurich for 2001–2004, carried out by a team headed by Susanne Fischer of the University of Zurich, showed that almost two-thirds of the cases of assisted suicide (64.6%) involved women. This skewed ratio, the authors of the study surmised, might be due to the fact that women tend to verbalize their feelings and seek help more often than do men. The large majority of individuals assisted (80.6%) were 65 years old or older. About one-third (34%) had been members of Exit for more than ten years; 24.5% had belonged for less than one year. (The membership numbers are not fully accurate; information about duration of membership was missing in 19.4% of the files.)[21]

During 2007, Exit had a team of 21 *Sterbehelfer* or *Freitodbegleiter* (assistants in suicide), an increase of six over the preceding year. The assistants are volunteers and receive compensation only for expenses. They play an important role because they visit the member who requests help, and they assess competence and other prerequisites for assistance in suicide. A senior assistant is in charge of the team.

As we have seen, in 1997, executive director Holenstein wanted to institute formal training for assistants, but at present it is not clear how much training assistants receive. According to a study published in 2007, approved volunteers "receive training in counseling, technical matters, and the policies and procedures of the organization and are subject to continuing education and supervision."[22] On the other hand, German journalist Svenja Flasspöhler, who actually observed the work of Exit for several months and published a book about her findings in 2007, notes that the assistants learn by doing—they observe the work of more-senior assistants a few times, then begin to function on their own.[23] From time to time, there has been talk about a more academic training program, but so far only a psychological examination to establish suitability, developed by the Institute of Applied Psychology, has been adopted.[24]

The team of assistants in suicide handled 287 new cases in 2007, of which 179 led to an actual assisted suicide—a rate of 62%.[25] Exit's yearly report, which includes these figures, does not break down this statistic. Some of the 38% of cases where no assisted suicide took place may have involved persons who changed their mind, some may have died of their disease before assistance could be rendered, and the requests of some may have been rejected. In an earlier report, then-president Schaer gave figures on accepted and rejected cases for 1996 (see Table 4.1).

These figures show that the acceptance rate for men was 93% and for women 80%, yielding a total acceptance rate of 86%. The report noted that the reasons for rejecting 14% of the requests was psychiatric illness or because the wish to die was inconsistent.[26] The Exit acceptance rate of 86% for 1996 is high when compared to the 37% of granted applications for euthanasia or PAS in the Netherlands in 1995.

Requests for assistance in suicide are reviewed by the head of Exit's department of assistance in suicide (*Abteilung Freitodbegleitung* or

TABLE 4.1 Disposition of Suicide Applications 1996

	Men	Women	Total
Number of applications	68	143	211
Applications approved by Exit-physician	63	114	177

Source: Undated Exit report (www.finalexit.org/swissframe.html).

Leitung FTB). During the last few years, two of these important Exit officials, Werner Kriesi and Walter Fesenbeckh, have been former ministers.
The decision to accept or reject an application is based on the applicant's
medical file, made available by the attending physician, and the report of
the assistant who visited the patient. The agreement of the family is considered important, but the patient's wish is decisive. In cases in which
unresolved medical, legal, or ethical issues are present, the final decision
is made by an Ethics Commission made up of a professor of legal medicine, an ethicist, two physicians, and three Exit officials.[27] We have no
data on how often this commission is involved in the decision-making
process or its rate of acceptance or rejection. The number of cases referred
to this commission is said to be small, about five each year.[28]

The Bosshard study found that 78.9% of the assisted suicides in
Canton Zurich involved patients suffering from fatal diseases such as
cancer, cardiovascular/respiratory diseases, human immunodeficiency
virus/acquired immune deficiency syndrome (HIV/AIDS), and neurological diseases. Seventy cases (21.1%) involved a nonfatal diagnosis such as
rheumatoid arthritis, osteoporosis, blindness, or general weakness.[29]
A more recent study, covering 2001–2004, showed that the rate of assisted
suicide for nonfatal cases had risen to 34.1%.[30] The granting of such
requests is in line with Exit's basic philosophy, which stresses the autonomy of the person and therefore sanctions help not only for terminal
patients but also for those with a serious disability or those who, for various reasons, are tired of life. Exit acknowledges that this involves "an
important step away from assistance to the dying to help in suicide."[31]
Exit members support this outlook and want to go even further. At a
meeting held in early 2007, it was resolved that, in order to safeguard self-
determination, a way should be found to obtain the lethal medication
needed for suicide without a physician's prescription.[32] Bosshard and
others, on the other hand, have expressed concern over whether the practice of helping persons without a terminal disease ignores or downplays
the availability of other therapeutic options.[33]

In its publications, Exit states that it supports palliative care, and in
August 1993, the organization opened its own hospice in the Villa Marga-
ritha located in Burgdorf (Canton Bern). It soon became clear that few
Exit members were interested in entering hospice care, and in 1995, the

facility closed.[34] Apart from this short episode, Exit records or publications show little evidence of palliative care being offered as an alternative to assisted suicide.

According to the Bosshard study, assisted death for persons with mental illness is rare. Out of the 331 cases of assisted suicide in Canton Zurich during 1990–2000, the wish to die was related to psychiatric disorders in nine cases (eight depression, one psychosis), a ratio of 3%. This number does not include cases in which the mental illness was present alongside a somatic disease. The number of strictly psychiatric cases has remained small even after the loosening of the moratorium on such cases in 2004. During 2005, out of a total of 162 cases, there we two instances of assisted death for psychiatric patients; in 2006, there were none.[35] In the yearly report for 2007, Exit reported that among the 179 cases of assisted suicide were one person with a psychiatric disorder and a second with beginning dementia.[36]

In psychiatric cases, Exit solicits an assessment from two psychiatrists, and each case is put before the Ethics Commission.[37] Still, much depends on the initial evaluation by the assistant in suicide, and a real question exists as to whether these individuals, without any kind of instruction in psychiatry, are able to ascertain the presence of psychic disorders such as depression—a difficult challenge even for physicians. An examination of an internal checklist kept by Exit assistants in suicide after 1998 showed that these assistants had identified the presence of clinical depression (*Krankheitsbedingte Depressionen*) in 27% of those cases for which the request for suicide was granted. The authors of the study publicizing these findings note that "because the persons conducting the screening are non-physicians, there may be a risk that a depressive disorder that impairs a person's decisional capacity could have been overlooked." Moreover, they add, "we do not know how much the Exit staff members were able to maintain the neutrality required for an objective assessment," rather than succumbing to overidentification with the applicants and thus minimizing issues likely to interfere with the receipt of assistance in dying. They surmise that an assessment of depression by a professional psychiatrist or psychologist most likely would have yielded an incidence of depression higher than the 27% identified by Exit staff.[38] The physicians who prescribe the lethal prescription theoretically could provide a layer of protection against a wrong assessment of competence. However, as discussed later in this chapter, since many of these physicians are sympathetic to Exit's strong endorsement of patient autonomy, this probably is a weak reed to lean upon.

Other findings raise similar concerns. An examination of the files of 43 patients assisted by Exit in Basel between 1992 and 1997 showed that Exit had paid insufficient attention to previous psychiatric disorders, including previous suicide attempts. The files did not indicate any effort to find solutions other than suicide.[39]

The expert assessment leading to the end of the moratorium had recommended that an interval of three months be observed between the psychiatric examination and any assistance in suicide. It also had suggested that one of the psychiatrists be from outside the Exit network of doctors.[40] Exit practice does not always conform to these recommendations. An internal evaluation of Exit's work found that, in handling the case of a member with serious psychological problems, Werner Kriesi, head of the department of assistance in dying, in 2004 had disregarded Exit guidelines and rules: To prevent a threatened suicide, Kriesi had provided the lethal drug to a person without remaining with that person. As it turned out, the person in question later changed his mind and is still alive. The case also led to a legal probe, which was still pending at the time of this report in early 2008.[41]

Many Swiss psychiatrists criticize Exit's approach to psychiatric illness and suicide as overly simplistic. The problem of suicide, they point out, is a complicated phenomenon that is yet only insufficiently understood. On the other hand, as Emile Durkheim stressed in his classic work *Suicide: A Study in Sociology,* societal attitudes to suicide and social position are an important factor. The elderly, for example, many of whom feel lonely and abandoned, have a suicide rate that is strikingly higher than that of younger people. There is concern that a right-to-die mentality will exert psychological pressure, especially upon vulnerable persons with serious psychological problems. Gerontopsychiatrists at the University of Bern hospital reported two cases in which psychiatric patients under treatment in the hospital, while on a short leave to visit their families, committed suicide with the help of a right-to-die organization (not clearly identified but is said to be Exit). Such patients may find in the ideology of such an organization support for their sense of despair and lead them to conclude that suicide is the only way out. While in the hospital and under the influence of doctors with a therapeutic approach, these patients had largely abandoned their wish for suicide.[42]

It is well-established that the desire to commit suicide among terminal patients fluctuates. It is therefore important to make sure that the wish to die is constant and that an adequate waiting period is observed between the request for assistance in suicide and the actual carrying out of the act. Exit is aware of this problem and stresses that the organization will generally not help individuals on short notice, especially those who join for the specific purpose of obtaining the immediate assistance of Exit. A membership of at least three months is the supposed prerequisite for obtaining help in dying, yet actual practice does not appear fully to conform to this rule. During 2007, the interval of time between the first visit by an assistant in suicide (*Erstgespräch*) and the act itself was seven days or less in 23% of the cases, and in a further 14% it was 8–14 days.[43] According to the Bosshard study, 10% of those assisted in suicide in Canton Zurich between 1997 and 2000 had been members of Exit for four weeks or less.[44] Svenja Flasspöhler notes that Exit sometimes proceeds too fast. In some cases, she writes, the decision to obtain the lethal drug is made during the assistant's first visit with the applicant.[45]

Exit members seeking assistance in suicide must have a physician's prescription for the lethal drug. In Canton Zurich, authorities require that this physician explicitly confirm the competence of such persons.[46] If a member's personal physician does not agree to write such a prescription, or if the member does not want to use this physician, Exit will refer him or her to a doctor sympathetic to Exit's goals (known as *Vertrauensarzt*—literally translated as a physician in whom Exit has confidence). The Bosshard study found that during 1997–2000, 31% of the prescriptions in Canton Zurich were written by the attending or family physicians, and 52% by an Exit physician (no information was found in 17% of the files).[47] According to a study involving cases during 2001–2004, the percentage of attending physicians was substantially higher (i.e., 61.9%).[48] It would be interesting to know how often physicians working with Exit reject such requests, but this information is not available. Bosshard and his co-authors expressed their concern over "whether the persistence of the death wish was tested adequately in those cases where the prescribing physician was not the attending or family doctor."[49] Exit doctors, they imply, can be expected to be more accommodating when evaluating requests for assisted suicide. One of these physicians, interviewed by Flasspöhler, told her that he does not like the label *Vertrauensarzt*, because it suggests that a doctor is working closely with Exit. At times, he stated, he does reject requests for the lethal drug.[50]

The desire for suicide sometimes is really a call for help, and the assurance of such help sometimes makes sick persons abandon their wish for suicide. The availability of a lethal drug often calms patients, and they eventually die a natural death. Once the Exit member has decided to go ahead, he or she decides the day of death. In the majority of cases (61% in 2001–2004),[51] the assisted death takes place in the member's home. Since January 2001, old-age and nursing homes in the city of Zurich allow organizations like Exit to assist patients in these facilities to commit suicide, presumably because most of these individuals have no other home.[52] The number of such cases is said to be relatively small. During 2007, 15 Exit members made use of the *Sterbezimmer* (dying rooms) maintained by the organization in Zurich and Bern.

The drug of choice is the barbiturate pentobarbital, which is brought to the place of suicide by the assistant in suicide. In 2007, the revelation that Exit maintained reserve portions of this drug in its Zurich office led to the confiscation of the stored drugs by Zurich authorities. Exit claimed that this reserve was needed in case of delayed delivery or spillage, although it was not explained how this reserve had been accumulated. An interim arrangement was eventually worked out that allows Exit assistants to carry a second portion of the drug.[53]

For patients who can no longer swallow, the lethal drug is administered intravenously, sometimes via a feeding tube to the stomach. During 2001–2004, this procedure was used in 24.5% of all cases of assisted suicide.[54] As long as it is the patient who opens the valve, the authorities accept this procedure as legitimate cases of assisted suicide. Minutes after ingestion, the person falls into a deep sleep. The time interval between oral ingestion of the drug and death is usually brief, 60 minutes or less in 88% of the cases examined in the Bosshard study. In at least one instance, the person seeking death continued to breathe for several hours, and the

Sterbehelfer resorted to a plastic bag to bring the dying process to an end. The daughter of this person reported the act to the police, and the Exit *Sterbehelfer* was brought to court in Zug and sentenced to a jail term of six months in early 2000.[55]

No serious complications or instances of reawakening from coma are known. The Bosshard study found that, in all cases, the authorities were duly notified.[56] Exit stresses the fact that it observes the law, takes pride in its good relations with the state, and indeed very few cases have ended up in court.[57] The organization also is on record stating that it would not object to further legal regulation of right-to-die organizations.[58] The current president of Exit, Hans Wehrli-Streiff, has said that he is in favor of legal regulation by the federal government.[59]

During 1990–2000, Exit assisted in the death of 748 persons, representing 0.1% of all deaths in Switzerland. By comparison, in Oregon, PAS under the Death with Dignity Act during 1998–2001 accounted for less than 0.1% of all deaths, while in the Netherlands euthanasia and PAS ranged from 2.7% of all deaths in 1990 to 2.2% in 2005. The number of persons availing themselves of Exit's assistance in dying has increased almost every year. It tripled between 1990 and 2000. In their 2003 study, the Bosshard team found that sociodemographic factors, such as age and gender, and medical factors (diagnosis) remained relatively unchanged. Since the quality of the records showed improvement (and, we may add, since the total number of suicides in Switzerland also did not change substantially during this period), they concluded that "this increase stems more from a growing number of requests than from relaxation of the indications for assisted suicide or from progressive laxity in decision-making."[60]

At his resignation as an Exit director in 2007, Andreas Blum charged just such a growing laxity. The data examined here suggest that the standards were never as high as one might wish. Among Swiss right-to-die organizations, Exit stands out as undoubtedly the most responsible. Yet, until action was taken by one of the Swiss cantons, its procedural safeguards were far from satisfactory.

Concerned about the unregulated practice of the canton's largest right-to-die organization, in the summer of 2009, Canton Zurich entered into an agreement with Exit that addresses some of the more important problem areas. Effective September 15, 2009, the aim of this agreement is to promote quality standards in the administration of assisted dying by the right-to-die organization Exit. To achieve financial transparency, the provisions include a ban on profit (Article 3.2.1), a maximum payment of Fr. 500 for expenses of assistants in suicide (Article 3.2.2), and the obligation to have Exit's financial statement monitored by a recognized auditor (Article 3.2.3). The agreement states that assistance in suicide is to be granted only to those "with severe suffering as a result of a disease," although suffering as a result of an accident or a serious disability is also included (Article 4.2). Those seeking assistance in suicide are to be provided with information about alternatives to suicide, such as palliative care, and a written report is to document the results of this discussion (Article 4.3).[61]

Several provisions of the agreement address competency and the constancy of the request for assisted suicide. To satisfy these criteria, the agreement calls for conversations with the person in question conducted "over several weeks" by the assistants in suicide and the treating physician and without the presence of next-of-kin or others who might exert pressure. The results of these conversations are to be included in the written report compiled by Exit. Exceptions to this procedure are possible in cases of a rapidly progressing disease, but even then a physician must examine the patient on at least two occasions (Articles 4.4.1, 4.5 and 6.1). Persons suffering from a psychiatric disease are to be examined by a psychiatrist, who must confirm that the desire to die is not the result of the psychiatric disorder. In difficult and questionable cases, two psychiatrists are to be involved. All such cases must also be discussed by the Ethics Commission of Exit (Articles 4.4.2 and 5.1.3). For patients with progressive dementia, competency is to be certified by two specialists in psychiatry or neurology or geriatrics (Article 4.4.3). In all cases, there must be a written certification by a physician detailing the nature of the disease and the competency of the person seeking assistance in suicide (Article 4.6.1). No assistance in suicide is to be granted to persons under the age of 25 who do not experience severe physical suffering (Article 4.4.4). Assistants in suicide in their first year are to consult with the head of Exit's department of assistance in suicide. The head of this department also decides whether a case should be discussed by the Ethics Commission (Article 5.1.2).

The person requesting assistance in suicide must take the initiative in contacting Exit. After all of the above-mentioned procedural conditions have been fulfilled and a physician has written a prescription for NaP (the only authorized medication to bring about death, Article 2), Exit must await a final request from the suicide seeker. This interlude gives the person in question additional time to affirm or reconsider the decision to seek assistance in suicide (Articles 5.1.1 and 5.1.6). Certifications by the involved physicians confirming that all required procedures have been followed are to be given to the police and the coroner (Article 5.1.9). Exit also commits itself to selecting assistants in suicide with care and to provide them with the requisite training (Article 7.1). An independent committee of at least three persons is to supervise Exit's practice in the provision of assisted suicide and to render a report to Exit once a year (Article 10.1).

The agreement between Canton Zurich and Exit is a first of its kind. It is to be hoped that at some early date Exit will allow a comprehensive examination of its practices in order to ascertain whether the regulations introduced by this agreement are being adequately implemented and whether they have successfully addressed previously existing shortcomings.

Exit—Association pour le Droit de mourir dans la Dignité/Suisse Romande

The second-largest Swiss right-to-die organization is Exit—Association pour le Droit de mourir dans la Dignité (ADMD)/Suisse Romande. Like Exit—German Switzerland, Exit of French Switzerland was also founded in 1982, but it operates independently of the German branch. The organization is headquartered in Geneva, and is open for membership to all residents of Switzerland above the age of 20, irrespective of nationality or religion. Annual dues are CHF 35. As of 2008, Exit—ADMD had 14,200 members.[62]

Exit—ADMD appears to follow more or less the same policies as the German branch, although we have far less information about its implementation of these policies or its mode of operation. Sandra Burkhardt, of the Institute for Legal Medicine at the University of Geneva, was given access to the files of the organization and, in 2007, published a study that provides some data for five years, from January 1, 2001 to December 31, 2005. The organization's bulletin often also includes some relevant information.

Both the number of requests and the instances of assisted death have increased sharply over the last few years (Table 4.2).

The difference between the number of requests granted and assistance carried out is accounted for by natural death, a subsequent change of mind, and cases pending at the end of the year. The rate of approval is higher than the already relatively high rate of approved cases at the German branch of Exit and is strikingly higher that the Dutch rate of PAS and euthanasia. We do not know who the physicians were who examined those patients seeking assistance in dying and who wrote the prescription for the lethal medication, whether they family doctors or physicians who were members of or close to Exit—ADMD. Burkhardt and colleagues report that, in 50% of those cases in which the files included a letter from a physician, the treating physician supported the request of the patient to die; in 31% he or she was opposed.[63] The data released by Exit indicate that despite the fact that nearly one-third of the treating physicians opposed the requested suicide, Exit granted more than 95% of all requests.

According to the Burkhardt study of Exit files, of the 200 patients who were helped to die during 2001–2005, 59% were women and 69% were over 70 years old. Ninety-five persons had cancer, 49 had neurological diseases, and 29 cardiovascular diseases. In line with Exit's philosophy, patients need not be terminal in order to qualify for help. During the period studied, 21 persons (10.5%) suffered from a multitude of disabilities that made them fear progressive deterioration and a loss of dignity, and they therefore decided to end their lives.[64] The situation of 21 of these

TABLE 4.2 Requests for Assisted Death and Their Disposition (2004–2007)

	Requests	Refused	Granted		Carried out
2004	158	6	152	96%	42
2005	202	4	198	98	54
2007	236	17	219	95	66

Source: *ADMD Bulletin*, no. 43 (2005), n.p., no. 45 (2006), p. 9, no. 49 (2008), p. 14.

persons is described in a study led by Maryam Zaré, who concludes that these were patients who could not be helped by palliative care.[65] Exit data for later years show a similar picture. In 2007, for example, 65% of those assisted to die were women, and 35% men. The average age was 75 years, with the youngest being 38 and the oldest 100 years old.[66]

As in German Switzerland, the lethal medication of choice is pento-barbital, preceded by an antivomiting dose. In 96% of the cases, the patient lost consciousness in less than 10 minutes. Death came within 30 minutes for 79% of the patients being assisted, although in one case it took 17.5 hours. More than 80% of the assisted suicides take place in the patient's home. In slightly less than one-third of the cases, a doctor was present.[67]

Most old-age and nursing homes in French Switzerland allow Exit—ADMD to provide assistance in suicide to their residents. The organization has sought permission to operate also in hospitals, and, unlike hospitals in German Switzerland, in 2006, the cantonal hospital of Lausanne (Centre Hospitalier Universitaire Vaudois or CHUV) agreed to this request. The hospital's policy requires meeting several criteria: Transfer to another institution or nursing home is not possible, the patient's illness must be in the terminal stage, and the patient must be fully competent to make the request for assisted suicide. The hospital also insists on an assessment by its psychiatric and palliative care service, although the final decision on whether to grant the request for PAS is made by an evaluations committee made up of a physician, a representative of the nursing administration, and two members of the hospital's ethics committee. The decision to allow PAS was taken over the objections of the institution's palliative care team, which was unanimous in rejecting the proposed acceptance of PAS and therefore does not participate in the evaluations committee that make the final decision. By June 2007, six patients had asked for PAS, but only one patient was actually assisted (two died before the review process was completed, one withdrew the request when the palliative care team was able to control his pain, and two applications were refused).[68]

In early 2007, the cantonal hospital of Geneva (Hospitaux Universitaires de Genève or HUG) likewise agreed to the request of Exit—ADMD for permission to provide PAS on its premises. Unlike the Lausanne hospital, HUG does not require a palliative or psychiatric consultation. On the other hand, staff members are prohibited from participation, and the assistance in death must be provided by a right-to-die organization such as Exit—ADMD.[69]

To have a full picture of the activities of Exit—ADMD one would need much additional information, but, as stated earlier, our knowledge of the organization's mode of operation is limited. We would want to know how Exit—ADMD arrives at its decisions in these difficult life-and-death situations, especially in instances in which the treating physician opposes granting the request for assisted suicide. Is there an ethics commission to decide especially difficult cases? What is the training of the assistants in suicide? How does the organization handle requests for assisted suicide from depressed persons or psychiatric cases in general? How is competency assessed? How persistent are the requests for assisted suicide, and how much time intervenes between the initial request and the assistance in suicide? How does the organization assess unbearable suffering, and does it draw attention to palliative care as an alternative to suicide? How many of the doctors prescribing the lethal medication are members of or close to Exit—ADMD? Full transparency would require answers to these kinds of questions, but so far we have no scientific study that addresses them.

Dignitas

In May 1998, a group of Exit—German Switzerland members, led by attorney Ludwig A. Minelli, quit Exit over the issue of excessive compensation for Exit's directors, and founded the right-to-die organization Dignitas. Located in Forch (Canton Zurich), as of 2006, Dignitas was said to have reached a membership of about 6,000 in 52 countries, with about 1,000 of these being residents of Switzerland. The two largest groups of foreign members lived in Germany (1,565 in 2004) and the United Kingdom (594 in 2004).[70]

In September 2005, Dignitas established a branch office in Hannover, Germany, but German members still must travel to Switzerland to avail themselves of the services of Dignitas. Members pay an initiation fee of CHF 100 and a yearly membership fee of at least CHF 50. Assisted suicide is charged at the rate of CHF 1,000–3,000 for Swiss residents and about CHF 3,500 for foreigners. In an interview with *Le Monde* on May 25, 2008, Minelli stated that during the ten years of its existence Dignitas had provided assisted suicide to 868 persons, the large majority of them foreigners.[71] The number of yearly cases has increased steadily. During 2001–2004, the total number for each year was below 100[72]; during the year 2006, on the other hand, Dignitas facilitated the suicide of 195 individuals, 120 of them Germans.[73]

The Fischer study of assisted suicide cases in the Canton Zurich during 2001–2004 showed that 91.2% of the persons assisted in suicide by Dignitas were foreigners, 21.2% of all cases involved a nonfatal disease, and 87.7% of those helped to die had been members of Dignitas for less than one year (13.2% for less than one month). The persons being assisted tended to be substantially younger than those handled by the German branch of Exit: 51.9% were below the age of 65 (vs. 18.4% for Exit), and only 5.8% were above the age of 85 (34.7% for Exit). Because of the large number of foreigners from countries where assisted suicide is illegal, 93.4% of the prescriptions for the lethal medication were written by Swiss doctors identified in the Fischer study as "physicians of the right-to-die organization."[74]

Because Dignitas provides assisted suicide to foreigners, and because it charges substantial fees, the organization has been the subject of much controversy. Critics charge Minelli with profiting from "suicide tourism" and with undignified ways of rushing seriously sick persons into death. Minelli has defended the practice of helping foreigners with the argument that he provides a needed service for seriously ill patients who cannot obtain relief in their own country, and with the argument that the European Convention on Human Rights forbids discrimination because of place of residence. As to financial rewards, he has stated that Dignitas merely seeks compensation for the large costs associated with providing assistance in suicide:– rent for the apartment where the assisted suicide takes place (and where patients coming from hospitals and foreign countries may have to stay for up to 2 weeks), the fee of the doctor who prescribes the medication, the expenses of the team of assistants in suicide, the death certificate registration fees, and cremation costs. About 80% of the members of Dignitas, Minelli said, never seek assistance in suicide because knowing that help is available makes them able to live with their fatal disease until natural death puts an end to their suffering. Those who do come to Switzerland are severely suffering patients for whom palliative care has not worked, and they demand quick relief. Dignitas, Minelli maintained, has to help quickly in these urgent situations.[75]

Information provided by persons who have worked for Minelli and media coverage tend to show that Minelli's account does not fully conform to Dignitas' actual mode of operation, and that the critics of Dignitas may have grounds for their fault-finding. One of the main reasons why Dutch law does not allow PAS or euthanasia for foreigners is because, in the Netherlands, physicians must know their patients before they can provide assistance in dying. Foreigners who come to Minelli's Dignitas, on the other hand, often are dead by the end of the day of their arrival in Switzerland. It would appear that these individuals receive only the most cursory examination by a physician who has never seen them before. According to Soraya Wernli, who for several years worked for Minelli, Minelli at times has used retired doctors no longer licensed to practice medicine. This charge is said to have been confirmed by Zurich public prosecutor Andreas Brunner.[76]

During the ten years of its existence, Dignitas has had many run-ins with various state authorities. Some have resulted from Dignitas providing suicide assistance to mentally impaired persons and, as of 2004, Minelli no longer accepts such patients even though he believes that the mentally ill have the same right to choose their manner of death as those mentally healthy. Minelli also has had difficulty finding psychiatrists willing to examine Dignitas patients.[77]

In several instances, residents of Swiss towns and villages have complained to the local authorities about Minelli's use of apartments in their houses as "death factories," and they have demanded the eviction of Dignitas and stricter enforcement of zoning regulations. In one such building, the number of assisted suicides had been so high that the residents called it the "house of horrors."[78] In July 2007, the municipality of Zürich-Wiedikon forbade the use of residential apartments for assisted suicide. Minelli thereupon moved his "dying room" to nearby Stäfa, but the authorities there similarly declared assisted suicide in a residential area a violation of existing zoning rules. In September 2007, it was reported that Minelli, running out of options, had started using his own apartment in Maur near Zurich. Several months later, he helped in the death of two Germans in a van stationed in a parking lot in a nearby forest.[79]

Minelli is on record as supporting the right of organizations like Dignitas to control the dispensing of the lethal medication used in assisted suicide. Because Dignitas has had difficulties finding physicians willing to write prescriptions for Minelli's numerous foreign patients, Minelli recently was reported to have started using helium gas, which is freely obtainable.[80]

Dignitas is organized as a society in which only Minelli and his two daughters are classified as active members. These three have the right to make all decisions. Since the actual assistance in suicide is provided by volunteers who receive no remuneration for their service, Minelli can earn a good salary as general secretary of Dignitas.[81] Faced with charges that he enriches himself through the practice of assisted suicide, Minelli repeatedly has promised greater financial transparency and outside auditing of the finances of Dignitas. One of the most recent such assurances of greater openness came in the summer of 2008, when Minelli told the *Basler Zeitung* that he will soon publish relevant financial data. Unfortunately, he added, he did not have enough time to follow up on this commitment.[82]

In March 2007, it became known that the Zurich authorities had started an investigation of Dignitas. The council of the Canton Zurich several times has voted on proposals to forbid "suicide-tourism" and even to outlaw the controversial organization. Some of these votes were close, but so far these motions have not carried. The much criticized mode of operation of Dignitas is one of the reasons why federal legislation to regulate the practices of organizations engaged in assisted suicide is given a good chance of approval. If this federal legislation were not to materialize, Canton Zurich may develop its own regulations. Such regulations are expected to include transparency with regard to finances, minimum professional standards for assistants in suicide, a waiting period between request for relief and the assisted suicide, and supervision of the physicians who write the prescriptions.[83]

Other Right-to-Die Organizations

In January 2002, the psychiatrist Peter Baumann resigned from Exit—German Switzerland over the issue of assisted suicide for mental patients, and, together with 27 other Exit members, founded the organization *Suizidhilfe* (assistance with suicide). Dr. Baumann had joined Exit in 1998, and between 2000 and 2001 had assisted in the suicide of 14 persons. Baumann's organization *Suizidhilfe* defends the absolute right of individuals to decide the timing of their death, including patients who suffer severely without a terminal somatic disease and are categorized as mentally ill.[84]

In early 2003, Baumann was arrested in Basel and charged on two counts—negligent homicide in two cases, and having assisted in another case "for selfish motives" because the assisted suicide had been filmed and subsequently broadcast on a television station. After having spent three months in custody, Baumann was released on condition that, until the end of the legal proceedings against him, he refrain from any further assistance in suicide. For all practical purposes, this meant the end of the organization *Suizidhilfe*. The subsequent legal proceedings are important, because they represent one of the few cases in which Swiss authorities have challenged the legality of a case of assisted suicide.

After numerous delays, Baumann's trial finally got under way in Basel on June 25, 2007. The psychiatrist was acquitted in one of the two cases of negligent homicide, but was found guilty in the case of the second person. Baumann had considered the individual in question competent, but the court, accepting the opinion of experts, rejected this finding. It concluded that Baumann had not acted with proper care in assisting in the suicide of an incompetent patient, and therefore was guilty of negligent homicide. In the case of the patient whose suicide had been broadcast on television, the court found that Baumann had acted out of a desire for publicity and that the assisted suicide therefore had taken place for "selfish motives," a violation of Article 115 of the Swiss criminal code. This finding was noteworthy because, until then, as Georg Bosshard notes, "the common legal understanding" had been that "selfish motives" had to do with "material benefits."[85]

On June 29, Baumann was sentenced to a jail term of three years, two of which were suspended. He also was ordered to pay the legal costs of the trial. Baumann appealed the verdict and sentence, and in late September 2008, the Basel Court of Appeal reaffirmed the finding of guilty in the case of the person with questionable competence and sentenced Baumann to a jail term of four years. On the other hand, the court acquitted Baumann of the charge of having acted for "selfish motives" when he had filmed an assisted suicide, thus restoring the previously prevailing identification of selfish motives with material benefits.[86] At this point, it is not known whether further appeals will be made in this case.

While the legal proceedings against Baumann were under way, the undaunted advocate of an absolute right to die in 2007 published a book *Suizid und Suizidhilfe: Eine neue Sicht* (Suicide and Assisted Suicide: A New View).[87] A reviewer in Exit—German Switzerland's newsletter called Baumann a zealot, who worked for greater freedom for the suffering individual but whose endeavors had the opposite effect, to whit, bringing about more controls and regulations that infringed on individual self-determination and autonomy.[88]

Another Swiss right-to-die organization is ExInternational, "Association for assistance in an autonomous dignified death," founded by Protestant minister Rolf Sigg. Between 1984 and 1997, Sigg had served as executive director of the German branch of Exit, but in 1997 he decided to establish his own organization. The aim of ExInternational was to expand assisted suicide to other countries and to help foreigners come to Switzerland to obtain this assistance. Several years ago, Sigg, who is now 92 years old, handed the leadership of the organization over to Zurich attorney Margrit Weibel.

Unlike Dignitas, ExInternational is a small organization that, for a time, attracted little public notice. The organization has a small staff and about 700–800 members in various European countries. There is no fixed membership fee, and members pay whatever they consider appropriate and are able to afford. Those of limited means can draw on a charitable fund maintained by the organization. Until the spring of 2008, ExInternational operated a small apartment in Bern, in which it assisted in the suicide of about 12 to 20 persons every year. Matters changed in 2007, when the activities of Dignitas led to negative media reports about "suicide tourism," and Ex International too began to encounter hostile comments from its Bern neighbors. In the winter of 2007, the organization therefore ended its work there and began to look for a new, more hospitable location.[89]

ExInternational stresses that it provides its services only after careful investigation. In a talk in Luxemburg in July 2006, Margrit Weibel described these procedures in the following way:

> On request for assisted suicide, the patient is visited several times by the respective assistant from ExInternational: (only travel expenses need to be reimbursed). A relationship of mutual trust and understanding grows as the assistant gets a clearer picture of the patient's medical situation, establishes whether the patient finds himself in an irreversible, mortal phase or whether he suffers of an unbearable physical condition without any hope of relief. It is equally important to establish that the wish to die has not been instigated by a third party.
>
> The patient must bring a doctor's certificate with the diagnosis of his situation; this is examined by a doctor in Switzerland, who will also make sure that the person is lucid and discerning.[90]

The founder of ExInternational, Rolf Sigg, several times got into trouble with Swiss and German authorities when he attempted to smuggle the lethal medication pentobarbital into Germany, and, in violation of German law, gave the substance to persons seeking assisted death.[91] Under the leadership of Sigg's successor, Margrit Weibel, the organization appears to have acted in conformity with Swiss and German law, and generally receives high marks for its professionalism. Still, the organization has published no data, and there exists no independent academic study of its mode of operation.

The Public Debate on Assisted Suicide

Over the years, the activities of the various Swiss right-to-die organizations have received extensive media coverage and have stimulated public discussion of assisted suicide. Public opinion surveys indicate that the Swiss public is broadly supportive of this practice, although the medical profession takes a somewhat more guarded view. Within these basic parameters, different surveys have yielded different results, a fact that is probably explained by the different wording of the questions asked.

According to a survey conducted in 1999, 82% of respondents agreed that "a person suffering from an incurable disease and who is in intolerable physical and psychological suffering has the right to ask for death and to obtain help for this purpose." Legislation to allow euthanasia was favored by 71%.[92] In October 2007, two surveys of Swiss public opinion conducted by the research institutes Demoscope and Isopublic showed that 53% of the Swiss population were in favor of allowing assisted suicide in desperate medical situations, and 54% expressed interest in personally availing themselves of this service. Only 15% supported a legal prohibition of assisted suicide. Assistance to foreigners, on the other hand, was seen more critically, with 54% opposing "suicide-tourism."[93] In 2008, a survey by the church paper *Reformiert* revealed that 75% of Swiss Protestants and 72% of Roman Catholics favored assisted death in extreme situations.[94]

The EURELD research project provides information on the attitudes of Swiss physicians toward assisted suicide. Based on data collected in 2002, 56% agreed with the statement "The use of drugs in lethal doses at the patient's explicit request is acceptable for patients in terminal illness with extreme uncontrollable pain or other distress." The rate of acceptance was highest in French-speaking Switzerland (65%) and lowest in the Italian region (41%). In the German-speaking part, the largest sector of the Swiss population, 53% supported PAS for terminally ill patients.[95] Another survey, conducted in 2006 and limited to French Switzerland, showed that 32% of doctors in that region had been confronted with a request for assistance in suicide and that 50% of these had responded favorably to this call for help in dying. Among those physicians who had never received a request for assisted suicide, 59% indicated that they could not envisage approving such requests.[96]

Swiss legislators, too, from time to time have discussed the issue of assisted death, although so far the results have been largely inconclusive. The Swiss parliament has only a small support staff, and most legislative initiatives therefore must come from the executive branch. In 1994, Victor Ruffy, a member of in the *Nationalrat,* the lower house of parliament (known as the "large chamber") proposed the decriminalization of euthanasia with safeguards, such as approval by two physicians. Two years later, after the motion had been changed to a postulate (a nonbinding resolution that merely called for a report), the *Nationalrat* approved the measure. In 1997, the Swiss cabinet, the *Bundesrat,* thereupon convened a multidisciplinary working group to examine the issue of assisted death.

The report of this group of experts from the fields of medicine, law, and ethics, the *Arbeitsgruppe Sterbehilfe*, was completed in March 1999. The working group agreed upon the importance of improving palliative care and on the need for legal regulation of assisted death, but failed to reach a consensus on how to modify Articles 114 and 115 of the criminal code.[97]

Several additional parliamentary initiatives took place in the lower house of parliament during 2000 and 2001 (introduced by Franco Cavalli, Dorle Vallender, Alexander Baumann, and Guido Zäch) without resulting in any action.[98] A resolution approved by both houses of the Swiss parliament in 2003 and 2004 called on the *Bundesrat* to propose legislation on assisted death, but the cabinet rejected the proposal on the grounds that the time for enacting new laws had not yet come.[99]

During the next two years, two prestigious professional associations weighed in on the subject of assisted death. In late 2004, the Swiss Academy of Medical Sciences (SAMS) issued new guidelines on the "Care of Patients in the Terminal Phase of Life." Whereas an earlier set of guidelines, published in 1995, had stated flatly that "assistance in suicide is not part of medical practice," the new rules, adopted by a different group of doctors, represented a more nuanced position. Patients in their terminal phase of life (defined as a situation that, according to experience, will lead to death within days or several weeks), the new guidelines stated, have a right to palliative care. The role of the doctor for these patients consists in alleviating symptoms; it is not his task to offer assistance in suicide. However, in some instances, the patient's suffering is unbearable and in these situations such a patient may express the desire for assistance in suicide.

In this special situation, the guidelines continued, the doctor faces a difficult conflict. On the one hand, assistance in suicide is not part of his normal medical practice; on the other, he is required to respect the wishes of his patients. In this dilemma, the physician must follow his conscience. He is not obligated to provide assistance in suicide, but his decision to do so must be respected. In that case, the physician must make sure the following preconditions are present:

- The patient is in a terminal phase of his illness.
- Alternative modes of treatment have been discussed and, if desired, have been implemented.

- The patient is competent, his wish for assisted suicide has been well thought out and is constant, and is not the result of outside pressure.
- The presence of these preconditions has been confirmed by a third person, although this person need not be a physician.

The final act leading to death has to be taken by the patient himself.[100]

Another important statement on the subject of assisted death was issued in April 2005 by the National Advisory Commission on Biomedical Ethics (NEK-CNE), a multidisciplinary group of experts in ethics, health care, law, and psychology that reflects Switzerland's linguistic diversity and includes a variety of ethical approaches. The commission has the legal mandate to advise the federal government and cantonal authorities on bioethical issues.

Opinion No. 9/2005 on the subject of "Assisted Suicide" recognized the conflict between the need to respect the autonomy of a person contemplating suicide and the requirement for society to provide care for such individuals so that the desire to commit suicide does not arise. Moreover, "the practice of suicide and assisted suicide must not restrict other peoples' freedom of choice, for example by making people who are disabled or sick feel that they cannot be a burden on society and must opt for suicide or assisted suicide."[101] There followed a set of recommendations, all but one either adopted unanimously or without dissenting votes.

The Commission proposed that, in accordance with Article 115 of the penal code, assisting in suicide without selfish motives remain unpunished. At the same time, the Commission took note of the fact that the law includes no provisions "concerning the protection of people at risk for suicide whose wish to die may possibly only be temporary and for whom other options may be available." Right-to-die organizations that help people to commit suicide, by their very nature, base their activities essentially only on respect for the autonomy of those wishing to commit suicide and neglect the need for counseling. The self- prescribed rules of right-to-die organizations are insufficient, since breaches of these rules by these organization—"which seem in fact to have occurred—are not subject to legal redress or sanctions. Therefore, the obligation to provide care for people at risk for suicide requires the introduction of new regulations making these organization subject to state supervision."[102]

Decisions on assisted suicide, the Commission emphasized, always had to be based on the individual situation of the person concerned. It was "essential to define certain necessary (but not sufficient) conditions and criteria, specifying when assisted suicide can legitimately be considered at all," as had been done in the SAMS guidelines. However, the decision to assist in suicide is always "more than merely a case of applying certain criteria and rules. It requires an in-depth knowledge of the person and the situation, the individual background to the desire for suicide, and the consistency of this wish. Furthermore, it requires prior discussion of possible alternative prospects, options, etc."[103]

For patients with a mental illness, the Commission stated, the desire for suicide is often a manifestation or symptom of their illness. These patients are in need of psychiatric treatment and psychosocial support, and assisted suicide for them is "generally ruled out." An exception to this rule "is the presence of a desire for suicide which is not a manifestation or symptom of the mental disorder and may occur for instance during a symptom-free interval of a hitherto chronic illness." If assisted suicide is allowed for such patients, it should not be carried out in psychiatric institutions whose function it is to treat mental disorders and their effect, such as suicidality.[104] For children and adolescents, a majority of the commission recommended special care to make sure that such patients "are in a position to assess their situation and prognosis fully and accurately." A minority came out against any assisted suicide for children and adolescents because it considered them as particularly prone to be influenced by external circumstances and other peoples' opinions. On account of their immaturity, children and adolescents were "especially at risk for impetuous suicidal acts" whereas in later life they may lose their wish to die.[105]

In the eyes of the Commission, it was the function of acute care hospitals and long-term care institutions to preserve and restore health, and to provide quality of life even at the end of life. It was not their task to bring about death; suicide in such institutions could create fears among patients and conflicts of duty. Still, the Commission recommended that if a resident of a long-term care institution had no other home, he or she be allowed to have the act of assisted suicide carried out there. In the case of acute care hospitals, the Commission suggested that such hospitals clearly specify whether assisted suicide would be permitted on their premises and take due care so that other patients not be affected. In all cases, a well-considered personal decision to commit suicide should not be frustrated by an institution's regulations or by the conscientious objection of an individual physician or an individual care team. "The option of being referred to another physician or transferred to another institution should be available if desired."[106]

The Commission stressed that it was the duty of health care professionals to foster life and not to help end it. If it were otherwise, and assisting in suicide formed part of medical duties, "every physician would be obliged to perform it when requested by a mentally competent patient." In cases in which physicians nevertheless assisted in suicide, they did so as a result of a personal decision. "Having made a decision for or against assisted suicide, as dictated by their conscience, health care professionals should not be subjected to moral disapproval or sanctions by their profession."[107]

As regards the problem of "suicide tourism," the Commission saw no ethical grounds for a general prohibition. The reasons for which nonresidents sought assisted suicide in Switzerland presumably were no different from those of Swiss people; hence, if one accepted in principle the moral legitimacy of assisted suicide, no justification existed for denying it to nonresidents. However, for this group, it was particularly important to ensure that adequate investigations into the condition of the patient and the consistency of his wish be performed. "For this purpose, a single, brief period of contact between the person's arrival in the country and the execution of the assisted suicide is generally not sufficient."[108]

The Commission noted the changing demographic structure of contemporary society as the proportion of older people increased and, with this, the number of those in need of care. A second trend was the rising cost of health care, particularly in the long-term care sector. The combination of these two social trends posed the risk of leading people in extreme situations to accept the organized provision of assisted suicide. In particular, older people with serious illnesses may develop feelings of guilt for placing a burden—financially and in terms of dependence on care—on family members, and this may lead them to the desire to commit suicide. The freedom and self-determination of those in need of care "could be jeopardized by the subjective feeling of pressure, on the one hand, and by the availability of socially accepted assisted suicide on the other—even if the people in need of care meet the criteria of mental competence and the right-to-die organization does not act out of self-seeking motives." The Commission warned that considerable attention would have to be paid to the prevention of suicide by providing care and support to the vulnerable, especially the sick elderly.[109]

The Commission's report concluded by emphasizing once more that "nobody can be entitled to receive assistance with suicide from a given person. Conversely, everybody has the right to refuse to assist a suicide, whoever they may be." This conscience clause was especially important for "health care professionals and members of staff in health care institutions. Assisted suicide is not one of the services that a patient can claim to be entitled to receive by virtue of the carers' professional skills."[110]

Opinion No. 9/2005, apart from a number of general indications, did not define those due care criteria for the practice of organized assisted suicide that should be specified in a supervisory regime. The Commission sought to fill this gap in Opinion No. 13, issued in 2006, that outlined duty-of-care criteria for the management of assisted suicide. The purpose of this opinion was to provide a set of minimum standards that organized right-to-die organizations were to uphold. The liberal legal situation prevailing in Switzerland with regard to assisted suicide, the Commission stated, created a need to protect individuals who wished to die with the help of right-to-die organizations. "The authorities have a legal duty to detect and investigate abuses. These efforts can be supported by ethical guidelines which clarify aspects that are crucial in specific cases from the viewpoint of protecting life."[111]

The Commission listed eight minimum requirements to make assisted suicide morally acceptable:

1. The patient must be mentally competent to bear witness and judge his situation. "It is important that the subjective view of the person desiring suicide should be decisive, rather than an evaluation according to extrinsic criteria."

2. Requests for suicide are to be considered only "from people suffering severely on account of illness." Assistance in suicide for those who are merely not satisfied with their life is ethically questionable. "While autonomy is a value of central importance, it is not the only value for organized assisted suicide."

3. Assisted suicide is not to be provided in cases in which the desire for suicide is a manifestation or symptom of mental illness. "In case of doubt, an expert should be consulted."

4. The wish to die must be enduring and constant. It should not be the result of an impulse or of a crisis of a temporary nature. An objective length of waiting time cannot be specified. The period of time to be required depends on whether there is the prospect of a change in the patient's situation and whether the patient has been able "to reflect adequately on the overall situation."

5. The desire for suicide has arisen in the absence of external pressure. Such pressure can take different forms: it can emanate from next of kin, be the result of financial difficulties, the sense of being a burden on relatives, etc. An assessment of whether a decision for suicide has been reached without external pressure requires individual discussions. "This rules out joint assessment of two or more people who wish to commit suicide together (e.g., double suicide of a couple). In such cases, there is a high risk that the initiative does not proceed from the two partners equally."

6. All options to alleviate the situation of the patient other than suicide (medical treatment, palliative care, etc.) have been explored, considered, and reviewed with the person requesting assistance in suicide. Whether to exhaust these other options is to be decided by the patient.

7. Repeated personal contacts and intensive discussions are required to assess the situation of the person desiring assistance in suicide. "This includes knowledge of the severe, illness-related suffering and information on the psychosocial context and biography, subject to the individual's right to respect for privacy." Such an assessment cannot be made on the basis of a single meeting or correspondence. "At the same time, the careful assessment should not be allowed to prolong the individual's suffering unnecessarily."

8. An independent second opinion, provided by a person with the necessary expertise, reaches the same conclusion on fulfilling the request for assisted suicide.

The Opinion concluded by stressing the need to prevent possible abuses within the right-to-die organization. This included lack of transparency in the mode of operation and management (including finances) or a lack of controls exercised by experts. The Commission probably had in mind the right-to-die organization Dignitas when it stated: "The risk is particularly high in the case of a nondemocratically organized association with a dominant leader, or a group with specific ideologically sympathies."[112]

The two NEK-CNE opinions represented carefully crafted position papers on assisted suicide. The Commission declared its indebtedness to the 2004 SAMS guidelines, but its position differed in one important aspect. Whereas the SAMS guidelines had limited assistance in suicide to patients in the terminal phase of their illness, the NEK-CNE position allowed such assistance in all cases of severe illness-induced suffering. This could include, for example, badly incapacitated and severely suffering patients with amyotrophic lateral sclerosis (ALS) who were not necessarily near death.

A more negative position on assisted suicide is held by the Swiss Association for Palliative Care (SAPC), a national organization founded in 1988. In November 2000, the organization sponsored a survey of its members on the subject of euthanasia and PAS. The survey showed that 69% of the membership—physicians, nurses, and other health care professionals working in palliative care—opposed euthanasia, and 56% rejected PAS.[113] In 2001, based on the results of this survey, the SAPC issued a position paper. In it, the organization regretted the inadequate attention paid to palliative care in Switzerland. The availability of palliative care was limited for the most part to cancer patients, and important differences existed among the various cantons. Hence, the organization concluded, until every terminally ill patient in the country had full access to palliative care, it was opposed to any attempt to legalize PAS or euthanasia.[114]

The public debate on assisted death reached a turning point by late 2003. In July 2003, the NEK-CNE had been requested by the Swiss Department of Justice to examine the ethical and legal aspects of the entire issue of assisted death, prepare a report, and develop proposals for legal regulation. The Commission had already independently started to consider these issues and continued with this work, according priority to assisted suicide. However, at the end of 2003, a newly constituted cabinet shelved this legislative project, and Christoph Blocher, the new head of the Department of Justice, withdrew his predecessor's request.[115] Blocher and his People's Party opposed assisted suicide and did not want the law to legitimize it. For the next four years, a tug of war continued between a widely articulated public demand for the legal regulation of assisted suicide as carried out by the right-to-die organizations and the equally strongly held view of councilor Blocher, who rejected any new additional involvement of the federal government in the area of assisted death.

Those demanding federal regulation of the right-to-die organizations pointed to the finding of the NEK-CNE study regarding the repeated violation of self-prescribed rules by these organizations. The state, wrote the theologian Ruth Baumann-Hölzle, has the obligation to protect the weak, and that required binding legislation along the lines of the SAMS guidelines.[116] Georg Bosshard suggested that the qualifications and training of those who carried out assistance in suicide was probably the most important area in which state regulation was needed. Beyond that, one might want to consider the registration and licensing of right-to-die organizations.[117] In November 2005, the prestigious and influential *Neue Zürcher Zeitung* called the absence of federal legislation regarding the activities of right-to-die organizations, especially with regard to the training of *Sterbehelfer*, "scandalous."[118]

In a lengthy position paper, released in draft form on January 31, 2006, Blocher's Department of Justice and Police explained why it opposed legislation that would regulate the activities of the right-to-die organizations. Overarching rules relating to assisted suicide were not practical because each case was different. The SAMS guidelines were adequate to regulate these decisions. The document acknowledged that the practice of the right-to-die organizations at times had led to abuses, but argued that these were due not to a lack of legal norms but to inadequate enforcement of existing laws. Any legal regulation of the right-to-die organizations would necessarily create a bureaucratization of assisted death, give these organizations added publicity, and provide them with official legitimacy. Their personnel, in effect, would become "officially licensed assistants in suicide."[119]

In as much as the lethal medication used in assisted suicide involved a narcotic (NaP), the position paper suggested that it might be possible to tighten the provisions of the law regulating the dispensing of narcotics. Changes in the law could obligate the physician to undertake a more thorough examination of the patient and require him to be present when the deadly medication is ingested. It was further suggested that one could also limit the availability of such medications to terminally ill patients or those without psychiatric problems.[120] Apart from changes in the narcotics law, the federation might also increase its contribution to palliative care. Beyond that, any regulation of the right-to-die organizations, including the problem of "suicide tourism," the document insisted, would have to come from the cantons and local authorities, rather than from the federal government.[121]

On May 31, 2006, the *Bundesrat* (cabinet) approved the position paper of the Department of Justice and Police and asked the department, in consultation with the Department of the Interior, to prepare concrete proposals with regard to changes in the narcotics dispensing law and for increased support of palliative care. When this report was issued in July 2007, it revealed that Blocher's negative attitude toward any regulation of assisted suicide had led to a retreat even in regard to the modest proposal for changes to the narcotics law. A more detailed regulation of the dispensing of narcotics, the new report now argued, violated the principle that such matters should be decided not by law but according to the recognized rules of the medical sciences. To require physicians to be present when patients consumed the medication, imposed upon doctors a "police" task that did not belong to the duties of the medical profession. Moreover, to supervise the work of physicians was the domain of the cantons and not of the federal government.[122] With regard to the promotion of palliative care, too, the report stressed the limited jurisdiction of the federal government and refrained from proposing any major initiatives.[123]

As expected, the cabinet also approved this second recommendation to forego new legislation with regard to assisted suicide. Although the right-to-die organizations were said to welcome this decision, much of the public reaction was more negative. The *Neue Luzerner Zeitung* noted that one could understand why the government did not want to "burn its fingers with the controversial issue of assisted suicide." Nevertheless, the paper wrote, the failure of the *Bundesrat* to act was "cowardly." The newspaper *Le Temps* remarked that the government, had avoided making a difficult decision by simply making no decisions at all.[124] According to a survey conducted in 2007, slightly less than a third of the Swiss population agreed with the way the cabinet had handled this issue, whereas 52% favored state regulation of the right-to-die organizations.[125]

The prestigious NEK-CNE also criticized the failure of the government to act. The president of the Commission, Christoph Rehmann-Sutter, joined by member Jean Martin, argued that the position of Justice Minister Blocher, embraced by the cabinet, ignored reality and made no sense. It was false to suggest that by regulating the right-to-die organizations one provided them legitimacy and assumed responsibility for their activities. Such a responsibility existed anyway, because of Article 115 of the criminal code, which enabled the right-to-die organizations to engage in assistance in suicide. At stake was the highest good—life itself. Should the state, the two NEK-CNE members asked, in order not to legitimize the traffic in weapons abandon the requirement that the possession of weapons required a permit?

The position paper of the Department of Justice and Police had maintained that the cantons had sufficient power to prevent any abuses on the part of the right-to-die organizations. In fact, Rehmann-Sutter and Martin pointed out, this assumption was contradicted by the testimony of the public prosecutor of Canton Zurich (the canton most affected by these abuses), who was on record stating that the existing laws did not allow him to investigate and punish existing misconduct.[126] Several months later, on October 29 2007, the *Kantonsrat* (cantonal parliament) of Zurich narrowly (by a vote of 80 in favor and 82 opposed) defeated a proposal to outlaw suicide tourism while at the same time it voted 94 to 56 to demand that the federal government enact the registration of and appropriate quality standards for the right-to die-organizations.[127] On June 21, 2007, the upper house of the federal parliament, the *Ständerat*, once again asked the government to propose legislation to regulate these organizations.[128]

A decision of the Swiss Supreme Court, handed down on November 3, 2006, strengthened the position of those who sought the government regulation of assisted suicide. The case involved a man with serious bipolar disorder, a member of Dignitas, who had been unable to obtain a doctor's prescription for the lethal medication NaP. The plaintiff claimed that, as an autonomous person, he had the right to end his life and therefore was entitled to obtain the medication through Dignitas even if no physician was willing to approve his request for assisted suicide. The court agreed that the plaintiff had the right to dispose of his life, but insisted that this right did not mean that the state had an obligation to help him in this endeavor. The regulation of the consumption of narcotics was part of the state's duty to protect the health and common good of the members of society, and a person's personal liberty did not give him the right to challenge the regulation of narcotics or any other valid state function. In principle, the court ruled, assisted suicide was not ruled out for a severely suffering patient with a psychiatric illness, although special caution was necessary in such cases. The responsibility for ensuring that patients were competent to request assisted suicide could not be put exclusively into the hands of right-to-die organizations. Some of the activities of these organization at times had given rise to criticism, and the state therefore was entitled to insist that patients receive a thorough medical examination—especially crucial for psychiatric patients—and that narcotics be dispensed only by physicians.[129]

The highest court in Switzerland had thus affirmed the right and duty of the state to regulate assisted suicide. Indirectly, but no less forcefully, the court had also given a green light to the state to regulate the mode of operation of the right-to-die organizations. The likelihood that such regulation would finally be enacted increased when, in December 2007, Christoph Blocher was not reelected as minister of justice. The new minister, Eveline Widmer-Schlumpf, made it clear that, unlike her predecessor, she is opposed to suicide tourism and sees the need for state action to guarantee certain minimum standards for right-to-die organizations. In an interview with the *Sonntags-Zeitung* on July 13, 2008, Widmer-Schlumpf suggested that there be an interval of time between the first visit to the patient and the act of assisted suicide. This would help limit suicide tourism. In addition, the minister proposed that right-to-die organizations provide full transparency about their finances, fully document each case of assisted suicide, and make public the qualifications of their *Sterbehelfer* who actually facilitate the act of suicide.[130]

The new minister of justice was not the only one to call for action by the federal government. In June 2008, the *Grosse Rat* (parliament) of Canton Argau voted to demand a ban on assisted death as a business, especially in the form of suicide tourism.[131] Not surprisingly, Dignitas drew further attention to the consequences of a largely unregulated regime of assisted suicide. As mentioned earlier, in order to circumvent the need of a prescription for NaP, Dignitas, in February 2008, started to use helium gas, which is available without a doctor's prescription. According to public prosecutor Brunner in Zurich, this involved putting a tightly tied plastic bag filled with helium over the head of the patient, who then died of suffocation. Dignitas had filmed several of these cases, and Brunner called the pictures "almost unbearable," for it took ten minutes for the patient to finally stop twitching. Minelli suggested that these were reflexes rather than conscious movements, and a director of Baumann's organization *Suizidhilfe* insisted that it took only one minute for the patient to lose consciousness as a result of the lack of oxygen. Brunner brushed these assurances aside and urged the federal government to act. The issue, he said, was not suicide tourism as such but clear rules of conduct for the right-to-die organizations.

Dignitas' use of helium gas was reported to have been one of the reasons why, in July 2008, the government finally appeared ready to undertake such regulation.[132] Minister of Justice Widmer-Schlumpf began to consult with moral theologians, ethicists, and prosecutors, as well as with representatives of right to-die organizations, and convened a working group to draft a proposal for the cabinet. Two such proposals to be considered by the Swiss parliament were announced by the *Bundesrat* on October 28, 2009. One of these options laid down strict rules of due care to be observed by those assisting suicide, while a second proposal involved a complete ban on organized assisted death.[133]

Under the proposal preferred by the government, those assisting suicide would commit a criminal offense unless they observed all the requirements of due care. To prevent impetuous decisions, those seeking aid in suicide would have to demonstrate a firm and constant wish for death, and a significant amount of time would have to pass before any action on such a request could be taken. Two doctors, independent of the right-to-die organization, would have to certify that the person wanting to die is legally competent to make such a request and that the suicidal individual suffers from a physical ailment that will result in death in a short time. Ruled out would be assisted suicide for those with chronic illnesses who are not in a terminal phase, or patients suffering from a mental disease. Furthermore, those assisting suicide must propose alternatives (such as palliative care), may not accept any payment that exceeds the actual expenses of the assisted suicide, and must carefully document each step in the assisted suicide to facilitate inquiries by the authorities.

The two best-known right-to-die organizations immediately announced their opposition to these proposals. Exit charged that the proposed regulations would in effect eliminate a patient's right to self-determination. Dignitas spoke of an incredible affront to chronically ill persons and those beset with mental problems, yet able to make rational judgments.[134] The Swiss parliament is scheduled to act on the two options by March 1, 2010.

5

PHYSICIAN-ASSISTED SUICIDE IN OREGON

The state of Oregon's Death with Dignity Act (DWDA) was a citizens' initiative, first passed by Oregon voters in November 1994 by a margin of 51% to 49%. A legal challenge delayed implementation of the law, but on October 27, 1997, the injunction against the legislation was lifted. After a ballot measure seeking repeal of the law had been rejected by the voters in November 1997 by an even larger majority than in 1994 (60% to 40%), Oregon became the first jurisdiction in the United States to allow physician-assisted suicide (PAS). The prolonged litigation that ensued after the passage of DWDA reveals the profound moral concerns raised by PAS in the United States.

A Legal Obstacle Course

Assisted suicide is prohibited, explicitly or implicitly, in practically all states. Until the enactment of Oregon's DWDA, and until the voters of Washington state approved the legality of PAS in November 2008, only three states—Massachusetts, North Carolina, and Vermont—had no statutory prohibitions against PAS or assisted suicide generally.[1] In the early 1990s, several physicians and their terminally ill patients in two separate actions brought suit demanding that the laws against assisted suicide in the states of Washington and New York be declared unconstitutional. The two cases, *Washington v. Glucksberg* and *Vacco v. Quill,* eventually reached the Supreme Court, and although the Court rejected a constitutional entitlement to assistance in suicide and upheld the two laws in question, it also left the states free to enact laws that would allow PAS.[2]

During the 1990s, the Hemlock Society provided much of the manpower and money for campaigns to legalize PAS. In Oregon, the Hemlock society supported bills allowing PAS introduced by State Senator Frank Roberts in 1987, 1989, 1991, but none of these bills became law. Similar endeavors failed in Washington, California, Michigan, and Maine, but did lead to the passage of the DWDA in Oregon in 1994. Fifteen days before the act was to take effect, on November 23, 1994, opponents of the law filed a complaint in federal court, alleging, among other things, that the law violated their equal protection rights under the 14th Amendment. After granting plaintiffs a preliminary injunction, the district court granted a permanent injunction against the enforcement of the law on August 3, 1995. The Court held that the DWDA did not apply equally to all citizens of Oregon, since it contained insufficient safeguards to prevent incompetent terminally ill adults from committing suicide. By depriving these vulnerable adults of safeguards available to other adults, the court held, the law violated the equal protection clause of the 14th Amendment. The plaintiffs' other claims were left unaddressed.[3]

On appeal, a three-judge panel of the Court of Appeals for the Ninth Circuit found against the plaintiffs on February 27, 1997. Without entering the merits of the dispute, the Court ruled on narrow technical grounds that the plaintiffs had not demonstrated an actual challenge to a legally protected interest and therefore lacked "standing" to file their complaint.[4] After a petition for certiorari to the U.S. Supreme Court had been denied, the Court of Appeals lifted the injunction on October 27, 1997.[5]

Oregon's DWDA had to survive several more challenges. A measure seeking repeal of the law was put on the ballot in November 1997, but the voters reaffirmed their support of the DWDA by the decisive majority of 60%. Opponents of the law now sought to use the federal Controlled Substances Act of 1970 to defeat it. After Attorney General Reno had voiced the view that this legislation was not meant to assign to the Drug Enforcement Administration (DEA) the role of resolving the profound debate about the morality and legality of PAS just because that procedure involved the use of controlled substances, Representative Henry Hyde and Senator Don Nickles sponsored the "Pain Relief Promotion Act of 1999" to amend the Controlled Substances Act of 1970. This bill sought to "prohibit the dispensing or distribution of a controlled substance for the purpose of causing, or assisting in causing, the suicide or euthanasia of any individual."

The bill did not become law, in part because of opposition from palliative care specialists who argued that this legislation would threaten legitimate pain relief. There was evidence to show that physicians, fearful of sanctions, already were prescribing less pain medications and patients reported increases in pain.[6] However, a new attorney general soon acted to accomplish what his predecessor Reno had held to be inappropriate.[7]

On November 6, 2001, U.S. Attorney General John Ashcroft issued a new interpretation of the Controlled Substances Act of 1970 under which assisting in suicide was held to be not a "legitimate medical purpose." The DEA was empowered to prosecute and revoke the DEA registration of any doctor who had assisted in a suicide in compliance with the DWDA.[8] On November 20, a federal district court issued a temporary restraining order against Ashcroft's ruling pending a new hearing, and this injunction was made permanent on April 17, 2002. The Department of Justice appealed this decision, and the case eventually reached the Supreme Court. On January 17, 2006, affirming the decision of the Ninth Circuit Court of Appeals, the Supreme Court ruled that the attorney general had exceeded his authority in interpreting the Controlled Substances Act to allow criminalization of conduct authorized by state law. The attorney general's authority to issue regulations for the control of drugs did not include the authority to define standards of medical practice.[9] Oregon's DWDA finally overcame its last legal hurdle.

The Death with Dignity Act

The law, which became effective on October 27, 1997[11], allows adult residents of Oregon (18 years or older) who are terminally ill to make a request to a physician licensed in Oregon for a lethal medication for the purpose of ending their lives "in a humane and dignified manner." (Physicians employed by the U.S. Veterans Administration are excluded.) The request must be made orally and in writing, be signed and dated by the patient, and be witnessed by at least two individuals, who in the presence of the patient must attest "that to the best of their knowledge and belief the patient is capable, acting voluntarily, and is not being coerced to sign the request." The oral request must be repeated not less than 15 days after making the initial request.

The physician who has the primary responsibility for the treatment of the patient's terminal disease must

- Determine that the patient has an incurable terminal disease that will produce death within six months, is capable (able to make and communicate health care decisions), and makes the request voluntarily
- Verify that the patient is a current resident of Oregon
- Ensure that the patient is making an informed decision by informing him or her of the medical diagnosis and prognosis, of the potential risks associated with the medication, and of feasible alternatives such as palliative care, hospice, and pain control.
- Refer the patient to a consulting physician for a medical confirmation of the diagnosis and for a determination that the patient is capable and acting voluntarily
- If either the attending or the consulting physician believes that the patient's judgment is impaired by a mental disorder, the patient must be referred to a psychiatrist or psychologist for an evaluation (such an evaluation may have to distinguish, for example, between an appropriate sadness or more pathological despair and depression)[10]
- Recommend that the patient notify his next of kin
- Counsel the patient about the importance of having another person present when the patient takes the medication and of not taking the medication in a public place
- Inform the patient that he or she can rescind the request for medication to end his or her life in a humane and dignified manner at any time, and offer the patient an opportunity to rescind at the end of the 15-day waiting period
- Dispense the lethal medication directly or write an appropriate prescription for a pharmacist (as of 1999, pharmacists must be informed of the prescribed medication's ultimate use, and

pharmacists in turn must report the prescribed medication to the Department of Human Services within ten days)

- Document or file in the patient's record the patient's oral and written request; his own and the consulting physician's diagnosis and prognosis, as well as the determination that the patient is capable, acting voluntarily, and has made an informed decision; the offer to rescind the request; and all steps taken to carry out the request, including a notation of the medication prescribed. A copy of this record is to be filed with the Department of Human Services.

The DWDA states that no person shall be subject to criminal liability, professional disciplinary action, or loss of privileges for good-faith compliance with this legislation. A conscience clause provides that no health care provider shall be under any duty to provide a patient with a medication to end his or her life, and any health care provider can establish a policy prohibiting such assistance on his premises. As an extension of this conscience clause, it also is not obligatory for physicians or pharmacists who are opposed to PAS to make referrals to other physicians or pharmacists.

The Department of Human Services is tasked to make rules to facilitate the collection of information regarding compliance with the provisions of the DWDA and to undertake an annual review of a sample of the records filed with the Department. The information obtained from physicians and pharmacists is privileged and may not be made available for inspection by the public. The Department is to create and make public an annual statistical report based on the information collected.

Under rules issued by the Department of Human Services, approximately one year from the publication of the annual report, all source documentation is destroyed. The Department checks on compliance with the provisions of the law and contacts physicians about missing or discrepant data. It also searches its Vital Records for death certificates that correspond to the reports by physicians. These death certificates make it possible to confirm patients' deaths and provide demographic information such as age, educational attainment, and the like. The Department also conducts follow-up telephone interviews with prescribing physicians to obtain information not available from the physicians' reports, including insurance status, enrollment in hospice, reasons for the request for a medication, and adverse reactions. Since the physician is not legally required to be present when the patient ingests the medication, the Department also seeks information from family members and friends who attended the patient's death in order better to understand patients' motivation for requesting PAS.[12]

Individual insurers determine whether to compensate patients for the costs of participation under the DWDA. Because of the federal Assisted Suicide Funding Restriction Act of 1997, federal funds cannot be used for services rendered under the law. The Oregon Medicare program does pay for these services, but only with funds provided by the state. The law provides that actions taken under the legislation do not constitute suicide, assisted suicide, or mercy killing and therefore do not affect insurance benefits by those definitions.[13]

A question that remains unresolved is how to handle the cases of patients who are qualified and capable of requesting the prescription for the lethal medication but are unable to swallow it. This problem may arise in the case of patients with amyotrophic lateral sclerosis (ALS or Lou Gehrig's disease). The law is clear in forbidding any individual to end a patient's life by lethal injection. However, suppose intravenous equipment is already in place for the treatment of pain or dehydration? Could this device be used by the patient to activate the delivery of a slow dose of the medication? A prescription for an "infusion" would appear to be clearly distinguishable from an "injection." The crucial requirement is that the medication, taken by whatever route, is self-administered.[14]

Even though patients with ALS have the highest rate of using the DWDA, to date only oral medications have been written. If a patient were to insist on obtaining a prescription for a self-administered infusion, it probably would then be up to a judge to decide whether the law (which does not specify how the medication is to be ingested) could allow for this mode of self-administered death.[15] The issue is also raised peripherally in a guidebook to the DWDA for health care professionals issued by the Task Force to Improve the Care of Terminally Ill Oregonians: "In making a decision to assist a patient with self-administering the medication, the health care professional [present] should be certain that the patient remains in control of the decision, timing, and every aspect of the action."[16]

Ten Years of Physician-assisted Death

The first yearly report on the implementation of the DWDA, for 1998, was issued by the Department of Human Services in February 1999. It showed that 16 Oregonians had availed themselves of the possibility of assisted death—0.06% of all deaths in the state during 2008. Since then, this number has increased gradually, reaching 49 in 2007, but even this represents no more than a tiny fraction of all terminally ill patients—0.16% of all deaths.

In early 2008, in conjunction with the passage of ten years under the law, the Department published a summary report for the 341 DWDA patients who had died after ingesting a lethal dose of medication during 1998–2007.[17] The data in Table 5.1 and the discussion that follows are taken from and based on this summary report. Important insights can also be gained from several independent studies of Oregonians who chose PAS undertaken during the years that the DWDA has been in force.

TABLE 5.1 Characteristics and End-of-Life Care of 341 Patients (1998–2007)

	Number	%*
Sex		
Male	183	53.7
Female	158	46.3
Age		
18–34	4	1.2
35–44	10	2.9
45–54	31	9.1
55–64	73	21.4
65–74	93	27.3
75–84	98	28.7
85+	32	9.4
Race		
White	332	97.4
Asian	6	1.8
Native American	1	0.3
Hispanic	2	0.6
African American	0	0.0
Marital status		
Married	154	45.2
Widowed	73	21.4
Divorced	86	25.2
Never married	28	8.2

(Continued)

TABLE 5.1 continued

	Number	%*
Education		
Less than high school	27	7.9
High school graduate	95	27.9
Some college	79	23.2
Baccalaureate	71	20.8
Postbaccalaureate	69	20.2
Underlying illness		
Cancer	280	82.1
Amyotrophic lateral sclerosis (ALS)	26	7.6
Chronic lower respiratory disease	15	4.4
HIV/AIDS	7	2.1
Heart disease	5	1.5
Other	8	2.3
End-of-Life Care		
Hospice		
Enrolled	291	85.8
Not enrolled	48	14.2
Unknown	2	
Insurance		
Private	212	62.9
Medicare or Medicaid	122	36.2
None	3	0.9
Unknown	4	
End-of-life Concerns		
Losing autonomy	300	89.0
Less able to engage in activities making life enjoyable	292	86.6
Loss of dignity	173	81.6
Losing control of bodily functions	196	58.2
Burden on family, friends/caregivers	132	39.2
Inadequate pain control or concern about it	92	27.3
Financial implications of treatment	9	2.7
PAS Process		
Referred for psychiatric evaluation	36	10.7
Patient died at		
Home (patient, family or friend)	319	93.5
Long-term care, assisted living or foster care facility	17	5.0
Hospital	1	0 3
Other	4	1.2
Lethal medication		
Secobarbital	175	51.3
Pentobarbital	161	47.2
Other	5	1.5

(*Continued*)

TABLE 5.1 continued

	Number	%*
Health care Provider Present when Medication Ingested		
Prescribing physician	74	27.9
Other provider, prescribing physician not present	140	52.8
No provider	51	19.2
Unknown	6	
Complications		
Regurgitated	19	5.7
Awakened after taking prescribed medication	1	
None	314	94.3
Unknown	8	
Emergency Medical Services		
Called after lethal medication ingested	4	1.2
Not called after lethal medication ingested	333	98.8
Unknown	4	
Timing of PAS Event (Median)		
Duration (weeks) of patient–physician relationship	11	
Duration (days) between prescription written and death	7	
Minutes between ingestion and unconsciousness	5	
Minutes between ingestion and death	25	

* Unknowns are excluded when calculating percentages
Source: Tenth Annual Report on Oregon's Death with Dignity Act (March 9, 2008)

The data collected and published by the Department of Human Services do not address all issues raised by the operation of the DWDA. For example, since physicians are not required to report the requests of patients who ask for but do not receive the medication, the published data do not show how many of these requests are refused. We do learn that about one-third of those who received the medication during 1998–2007 did not use it and eventually died of natural causes (see Table 5.2). In some cases, receipt of the medication may have come too late, although this fact is unlikely to explain all cases. The knowledge that they were in full control of the dying process apparently provided enough reassurance for large numbers of patients to abandon their planned suicide.

Before the enactment of the DWDA, concerns had been voiced that PAS would be chosen by a disproportionate number of poor and uneducated patients. The data available show that these fears were unfounded.

TABLE 5.2 Prescription History under the Death with Dignity Act

Year	Prescriptions filled	Deaths	Percentage of prescriptions used
1998	24	16	67
1999	33	27	82
2000	39	27	69
2001	44	21	50
2002	58	38	66
2003	68	42	62
2004	60	37	62
2005	65	38	58
2006	65	46	71
2007	85	49	58
		Average used	65%
		Average not used	35%

Source: Tenth Annual Report on Oregon's Death with Dignity Act (March 9, 2008)

Compared with other Oregon residents who died between 1998 and 2007, those who chose PAS were more likely to be better educated. Education was found to be the demographic variable most strongly related to reliance upon the law. As many as 41% who died under the DWDA had college or graduate degrees, whereas only 15% of all persons who died of other causes during these years had this higher level of education.

The data collected by the Department of Human Services do not include income level, but an independent study showed that those with higher incomes were more likely to make use of or consider PAS.[18] Moreover, education is known to be a good substitute for income. Thus, it is clear that poor people did not disproportionately end their lives through PAS. Being a burden on family and friends was cited as a concern by close to half of those who relied upon the law, but since only 2.7% of those who used the DWDA cited the financial implications of treatment as an end-of-life concern, the burden they were worried about apparently was not monetary. The financial costs of illness represented the least important of the different concerns mentioned. All Oregonians dying under the DWDA had insurance.[19]

Other demographic characteristics similarly are not associated with greater use of the DWDA. Women and older people were thought to be groups vulnerable to pressures to hasten their death, but there is no evidence that this is the case. During ten years of the law's operation, more men (53.7%) than women (46.3%) chose PAS, and the very old, those above the age of 84, are under-represented among those using the law. The same holds true for members of minority groups such as Blacks, Hispanics, and Native Americans.

Divorced and never married persons did make use of PAS in disproportionately larger numbers. The reasons for this finding are not entirely clear, but may have to do with the weaker social network these persons have in comparison with married couples. The divorced and never married probably receive less assistance from family and friends at a time when terminally ills persons need help with such things as home care and transportation. The divorced and never married may also have fewer family concerns—they do not have to worry about the welfare of a spouse or about the impact of their suicide upon their spouse.[20]

The most frequently cited reason for choosing PAS was the fear of losing control and autonomy. The inability to engage in enjoyable activities, loss of dignity, and no longer having control of bodily functions were also among the primary factors contributing to patients' requests for assistance in dying. Many of these patients did not wait until they were bedridden to end their lives, thus indicating a pronounced desire to control the manner and time of their death. Doctors characterized these persons as strong and forceful personalities: "Many of the physicians who prescribed a lethal medication reported that their patients had been decisive and independent throughout their lives or that the decision to request a lethal prescription was consistent with a longstanding belief about the importance of controlling the manner in which they died." Hospice chaplains, hospice nurses, and hospice social workers concurred with this assessment, stating that being in control and remaining independent was among the most important reasons for patients seeking PAS. Although some patients do change their minds about assisted suicide after receiving improved palliative care, for strong personalities the very thought of more care may be unacceptable because it involves more dependence. Those for whom religion is not very important were also more likely to choose assistance in dying.[21]

Inadequate pain control or concern about it was cited only by one-third of all those making use of the DWDA. In fact, a substantial number of hospice nurses reported that patients seeking PAS had less pain than other hospice patients.[22] Oregonians, it appears, do not make use of the DWDA because of lack of good end-of-life care. Since the enactment of the law, enrollment in hospice has increased steadily, and it is now the highest in the nation. In 1994, 22% of all deaths in Oregon occurred in persons enrolled in hospice. By 2007, 88% of all those choosing PAS were being cared for by hospice, and in 2008, this percentage reached an all-time high of 98%.[23] By 2007, 90% of deaths under the DWDA took place at home, where most patients prefer to die, the highest rate in the United States. Oregon also has the lowest rate of hospital deaths. Family members mentioned improved pain management after entering hospice care, and, according to one study, one out of three patients who had intended to choose PAS in 2004 changed their mind after receiving good palliative hospice care.[24] In 2007, the Oregon Hospice Association noted with pride that the relatively low rate of Oregonians opting for assisted death is a reflection of the high quality of care provided by Oregon Hospice.[25]

The Oregon Hospice Association had opposed the DWDA in 1994 and 1997, but since then has accepted PAS as a legal option. "Oregon's Death with Dignity Act," the association noted in 2006, "has been responsibly implemented with none of the predicted dire consequences."[26] In a survey of Oregon physicians carried out in 1999, 13% stated that since passage of the DWDA they had become more favorably disposed toward the law, but only 51% indicated their support of the DWDA, 31% were opposed, and 17% considered themselves neither supportive nor opposed. About one-third of these physicians (34%) were willing to prescribe a lethal medication in accordance with the DWDA, 20% were uncertain, and 46% were unwilling to do so.[27] No other survey of Oregon physicians has been carried out since 1999, and we therefore do not know whether Oregon doctors since then have become less sharply divided in their attitude toward the DWDA.

Physicians who have prescribed a lethal medication under the law report that it involved a large emotional investment and a highly intense experience, similar to the reaction of Dutch doctors we mentioned in

Chapter 2. Still, beliefs that their actions were "the right thing to do" usually overrode feelings of discomfort. Physicians also noted that "going through with the assisted suicide decision-making process had a positive impact on them personally, and on their ability to speak with patients about the end of life." Not knowing patients made decision-making harder, whereas having known the patient for a long time made it easier to deal with the request of assisted suicide. In most cases, physicians felt that things had gone well; that is, "deaths seemed peaceful, rapid, and allowed time for patients to spend time with families." Physicians from rural communities, where the issue of PAS is more controversial and there is less physician anonymity, reported fears that involvement in assisted suicide would affect their reputations, ability to maintain practices, or relationships with colleagues or partners.[28] A fear of ostracism by patients and colleagues on the part of some physicians has been relayed also by another investigator earlier in the history of the DWDA.[29]

The 1999 survey of Oregon physicians shows that physicians who received requests for a prescription for the lethal medication were somewhat more favorably disposed toward the DWDA and were significantly more willing to write a prescription (51% vs. 34% of all physicians). Still, these doctors approved only 18% of the requests received (about 1 in 6), and only about half of these (59%) actually resulted in a suicide (about 1 in 10).[30] The 18% rate of approved requests is low when compared with the Dutch rate of approval for euthanasia and PAS, which was 37% in 1995. In 1999, physicians handling request for PAS from members of the right-to-die organization Exit in German-speaking Switzerland approved 86% of all such requests. Altogether, in 1999, PAS was involved in 0.1% of all deaths in Oregon.[31] By contrast, PAS was the cause of 0.36% of all deaths in Switzerland. In other words, assisted death in Switzerland involved the deaths of more than three times as many persons as in Oregon.

In contrast to the sharply divided medical community, Oregon hospice nurses and social workers working in in-home hospice programs display a more favorable attitude toward the DWDA. A survey conducted in 2001 showed that, on an attitude scale with a range of 1 (completely disagree) to 5 (completely agree), nurses and social workers had a score of 3.4 and 3.9 respectively. Large numbers of nurses and social workers in

hospice work apparently do not see hospice and PAS as mutually exclusive alternatives. Only 5% thought that patients who wanted assisted suicide should be discharged from hospice.[32]

Prior to the 1994 election, when PAS first appeared on the ballot of
Oregon voters, the House of Delegates of the Oregon State Pharmacists
Association (OSPA) voted unanimously to oppose the DWDA. Pharmacists resented not having been consulted in the drafting of the initiative.
Moreover, as they saw it, they had been educated in the healing arts to
prolong life, rather than to shorten it. Following the approval of the law,
OSPA stated that it would work with the Oregon Board of Pharmacy to
establish protocols for the lethal medications used, so that it could carry
out the will of the electorate.[33]

Based on these protocols, according to the 2008 summary report on
ten years of the DWDA, practically all physicians have prescribed the barbiturates secobarbital or pentobarbital, usually preceded by a medication
to prevent vomiting. No complications were reported in 94.3% of the
cases. The median time between ingestion of the medication and losing
consciousness was 5 minutes, and 25 minutes elapsed between ingestion
and death. In 19 cases (5.7%) patients regurgitated some of the medication. In 2005, one patient regained consciousness 65 hours after ingesting
the medication, and subsequently died from the underlying illness two
weeks after awakening. Under the Oregon Act, physicians are not permitted to provide a lethal injection if the patient's self-administered medication does not result in death.[34]

In the Netherlands, the Regional Review Committees have recommended that physicians providing assisted suicide stay with their patients
until death occurs. In the case of complications, such as vomiting of the
medication, they can use an injection to bring about death. This option is
not available to Oregon physicians; neither are they required to be with
the patients for whom they have prescribed the lethal medication. During
the ten years of the DWDA, prescribing physicians were present when
their patients took the medication in only 28% of the cases. In 53% of the
instances of PAS, someone other than a doctor attended the patient. The
right-to-die organization Compassion and Choices is said to have provided volunteers to be with such patients during their final hour in three-
quarters of all cases of PAS.[35]

Because of the possibility of complications, ethicist Raphael Cohen-Almagor has suggested that, as in the Netherlands, physicians accompany their patients in this last step.[36] If the prevention and relief of suffering are the aims of medical interventions, physician-author Sherwin B. Nuland has written, physicians should be present during an assisted suicide in order "to ensure that death is as merciful and serene as possible."[37] Still, as Oregon data show, most physicians prefer not to comply with this advice. Unlike in the Netherlands, American doctors are not necessarily acquainted with their patients for a very long time. The data indicate that the median duration of the physician–patient relationship in Oregon cases of PAS was no more than 11 weeks. Hence, many doctors lack the motivation to go out of their way for these patients; their relationship with the patient having been relatively short, they also may hesitate to intrude upon the family and friends who often accompany their loved ones in this final act.

Emergency Medical Services were called in four cases (1.2%) of death under the DWDA, although none of these patients called for intervention after ingestion of the lethal medication. If such a call were to occur, emergency medical staff, in order to protect patient autonomy, are expected to ascertain why 911 was called, and whether the person no longer wishes end his or her life. They also are to respect Do Not Attempt Resuscitation (DNAR) requests. Oregon has a high rate of Physician Orders for Life Sustaining Treatment (POLST) forms that enable health care professionals to honor the end-of-life treatment desires of patients.[38]

Criticism and Problem Areas

As in other countries where PAS is legal, enforcement of the provisions of the DWDA is dependent upon the self-reporting of physicians, with all the obvious problems that such a system entails. A study undertaken at the behest of the Health Division of the Oregon Department of Human Services and published in 2000 acknowledged: "Under-reporting cannot be assessed, and noncompliance is difficult to assess because of the possible repercussions for noncompliant physicians reporting data to the division."[39] On the other hand, the rule introduced in 1999, requiring pharmacists to report the dispensing of lethal medications within ten days, should make it much easier to detect instances of doctors failing to report PAS. Rules of medical practice issued by the Oregon Board of Medical Examiners also make it mandatory for licensed physicians to report the unprofessional conduct of another doctor within ten working days, and that obligation includes reporting noncompliance with DWDA safeguards. Failure to report a fellow licensee may result in disciplinary action against the professional who knew of the inappropriate or illegal conduct.[40]

The conclusion of John Keown, a well-known opponent of any type of assisted death, that the reporting system of the DWDA is entirely useless, would therefore appear to be overly broad.[41] Adherence to most standards of proper medical practice, including decisions not to start or to forego life-sustaining treatment, similarly depends on the professionalism of doctors rather than on strict control of noncompliance by the state. A study of professionalism in medicine published in 2007 concluded that, although many physicians fell short in such matters as reporting impaired or incompetent colleagues or in managing financial conflicts of interest, most doctors reported a high level of conformity with the most important tenets of professional conduct.[42]

The criticism by Kathleen Foley and Herbert Hendin, two other opponents of PAS, that the DWDA lacks "enforcement mechanism," also is not accurate.[43] Although the Oregon Health Division is not a regulatory agency for physicians and is not assigned enforcement authority, it does report any cases of noncompliance to the appropriate state agency. In 2001, for example, a doctor who had submitted an incomplete written consent was reported to the Board of Medical Examiners.[44]

John Keown has noted that "a significant proportion of patients 'shop around' to find a compliant doctor," and has cited this as another weakness of the law.[45] In view of the fact, noted above, that a substantial segment of the medical community is opposed to the DWDA and is unwilling to write a prescription for a lethal medication, the frequent need of patients to have to ask more than one physician is to be expected. Sullivan and his co-authors report that only 31% of patients received a prescription from the first doctor they asked, and some had to ask two or three doctors.[46] It is also no secret that the right-to-die organization Compassion and Choices helps patients find doctors who in principle are prepared to write prescriptions. Reflecting this referral process, 27% of physicians surveyed in 1999 who had received a request for a prescription had known the patient for less than one month at the time of the request for assistance with suicide.[47]

The summary report of the Department of Human Services for 1998–2007 shows that during these ten years, 294 physicians wrote a total of 541 prescriptions, with the average number per doctor being 1.7 prescriptions. These 294 doctors constitute 3.4% of all Oregon physicians.[48] Can doctors supportive of the DWDA be expected to be rigorous in adhering to the provisions of the law, or is their performance similar to that of the Swiss *Vertrauensärzte* (physicians in whom Exit has confidence) who almost routinely approve most requests for PAS? The fact, mentioned earlier, that in Oregon, according to 1999 data, the approval rate for assistance in suicide was only 18% (or about 1 in 6) would seem to indicate that these physicians do indeed adhere to the requirements of the Oregon law.

John Keown has called the DWDA "the most permissive regime for PAS yet devised" in part because there is no requirement that the patient be suffering "let alone be suffering severely and unbearably," as in the Dutch and Belgian legislation.[49] Keown is correct that the Oregon law does not make suffering a requirement for PAS, but the DWDA is available only to terminally ill patients and that probably is a far more restrictive provision (absent from both the Dutch and Belgian law). It excludes, for example, nonterminal patients with degenerative neurological diseases such ALS. Moreover, "suffering" is a largely subjective criterion, whereas the presence of a terminal condition is a matter of empirical determination. It also is unlikely that very many terminal patients will opt for PAS unless they are suffering severely. Even if a terminal patient is not yet suffering acutely, concern, not to say fear, of suffering that lies ahead may itself induce severe distress.

The 1999 survey of Oregon physicians undertaken by Ganzini and colleagues had shown that "one in six were not confident about finding reliable lethal prescribing information, and one in four were not confident in determining six-month life expectancy."[50] However, during the following years, competency in terminal care has undoubtedly improved considerably. In May 1995, an expanded curriculum in comprehensive end-of-life care was implemented at Oregon Health Sciences University.

Several Oregon hospitals have developed or expanded interdisciplinary teams to function as consultants in comfort care.[51] By 2007, as we have seen, 88% of those who died under the DWDA were under hospice care.

The Assisted Suicide Consensus Panel, part of the Finding Common Ground Project of the University of Pennsylvania Center for Bioethics, has publicized suggestions for improved communication with terminal patients and on how to respond to those who request PAS.[52] There is reason to think, concludes Timothy Quill, that these various efforts, in addition to the effects of legalization itself, have resulted in more open conversation about end-of-life options.[53]

And yet, to ensure the availability of palliative care for everyone, it might be desirable if the consulting physician were to be an expert in palliative care, similar perhaps to the Support and Consultation in the Netherlands (SCEN) program or the palliative filter used by Caritas in Belgium. The need for such monitoring by someone with expertise in end-of-life care is stressed not only by opponents of PAS, such as Kathleen Foley, Herbert Hendin, and Neil Gorsuch, but also by proponents like Linda Ganzini.[54]

The difficulty of recognizing psychiatric disorders such as clinical depression is another problem not fully solved by the Oregon DWDA. The law requires that, if either the attending or the consulting physician suspect a mental disorder that could impair the judgment of the patient requesting a prescription for a lethal medication, the patient be referred to a mental health practitioner for an evaluation. But can one be sure that ordinary physicians will recognize the need for such a consultation? Many of them, it has been suggested, may consider a depressive mood in terminal cases as normal.[55]

During the ten years of the DWDA, only 36 patients (10.7%) were referred for a psychiatric consultation, and during 2007, there were no referrals at all. According to studies of patients who died under the law, the number of actual cases of depression is likely to have been higher. "Our study suggests," conclude Linda Ganzini and her co-authors in an article published in 2008, "that in some cases depression is missed or overlooked," and current DWDA practice therefore "may allow some potentially ineligible patients to receive a prescription for a lethal drug."[56] This conclusion is in line with other research, discussed in our introductory chapter, that indicates that physicians who are not psychiatrists under-diagnose depression.[57] A study of oncologists published in 1998 revealed that these physicians accurately diagnosed only 20 (13%) of 159 moderately to severely depressed patients and rated 78 (49%) of these patients as essentially having no depressive symptoms.[58]

Even a psychiatric examination does not provide assurance that competency can be established in a reliable manner. Ganzini and her team found that only 6% of Oregon psychiatrists were confident that, in a single evaluation, they could adequately determine whether a psychiatric disorder was impairing the judgment of a patient requesting PAS.[59] Many psychiatrists therefore recommend that the presence of a major depression should result in an automatic finding of incompetence for the purpose of obtaining assisted suicide. Ganzini and colleagues suggest a mental health consultation and a systematic examination for depression for all patients seeking PAS.[60] The Task Force to Improve the Care of Terminally Ill Oregonians, in its 2007 report, similarly recommended a mental health consultation for any person desiring a prescription under the Act. Such an examination was especially important for patients not in hospice care.[61]

The issue of a "psychiatric filter" so far has remained unaddressed, and the absence of such an obligatory psychiatric consultation in the eyes of some constitutes a serious shortcoming of the DWDA. Another problem is the limitation of the law to adult patients. A 1998 survey of oncologists, including pediatric oncologists, revealed that oncologists handling minors resorted to PAS and euthanasia at rates far higher than adult oncologists. For example, whereas 3.7% of adult oncologists reported to have performed euthanasia for between one and five patients, the rate was 8.6% for pediatric oncologists.[62] Terminal children, it would appear, are involved in these difficult life-and-death dilemmas far more frequently than adult patients, and therefore a clear need exists to provide guidelines for the care of these children.

Also not dealt with by the law is the problem of extremely premature or low-birthweight babies. During the past three decades, neonatal mortality has been reduced sharply, but the outcome for some of these babies is still poor. The situation in these cases is complicated by the fact that neonates, unlike even young adults, cannot make decisions, express their views, or write a living will. Called into question are medical circumstances that might justify euthanasia to spare the child life-long pain and suffering. Death, everyone agrees, is not the only bad outcome to be avoided. But to what extent may predictions of quality of life enter into these decisions? Questions also arise with regard to who is entitled to make decisions on behalf of these babies—parents for whom the consequences matter most, or pediatricians acting as advocates in the child's "best interests."[63]

The issue of what constitute the "best interests" of a child in these complex situations is addressed by guidelines issued by the Academy of Pediatrics in 1994. Prolonging life will usually be in the best interest of the unfortunate child, provided it is not excessively burdensome or disproportionate in relation to expected benefits. The "best interests" standard, the guidelines declare, involves balancing the benefits and burdens of present and future treatments, an assessment of the present and future quality of life (including physical pleasure or irremediable disability, emotional enjoyment or suffering), and the futility of present treatment.[64]

Physicians are not required to provide futile care, but the determination of futility is often far from easy, and many of these assessments turn out to be inaccurate. William Meadows, director of a neonatal intensive care unit (NICU) in Chicago, studied the predictions of health care professionals in his unit and found that even when every one of several caretakers predicted that a certain infant would die within three days in a row, they were wrong 18% of the time. The stakes in these cases are high, for the greater the risk of death, the greater the risk of survival with serious impairment. Meadows and Lantos concluded that decisions to withhold or withdraw treatment could not be based on the certainty of futility, and that such decisions necessarily had to be based on probabilistic information about outcomes.[65] The Oregon DWDA does not deal with these dilemmas and provides no legal guidance in this difficult area of medical care.

Experience with the DWDA, one observer has concluded, has been "for the most part reassuring: medical and legal safeguards established during implementation appear to have prevented abuse, and most patients have had the expected outcome." Some may disagree with this assessment, but even this student of the subject has acknowledged that

"Oregon's successful implementation of its assisted-suicide law might not be easily replicated in other states with more socioeconomically diverse populations and less inclusive health care programs." There is a limited demand for assisted suicide in a system with good care, such as Oregon's, but there might be far larger demand for PAS in a state with much less adequate care.[66]

6

ASSISTED DEATH AS A LAST RESORT

In a book of essays, published in 1998, Paul van der Maas and Linda L. Emanuel called for more empirical research into the various ethical, medical, and legal issues surrounding the practice of physician-assisted suicide (PAS). "It is our belief," they wrote "that new empirical studies will greatly improve the quality of the ethical debate both in society generally and in the profession, will assist in the formulation of responsible public regulations, will promote and guide the quality of medical training, and, most importantly will help improve the quality of care for the dying."[1] Some ten years later, much of this expectation has been fulfilled. The four regimes of PAS and euthanasia now functioning have been studied extensively and can provide significant lessons concerning the practice of assisted death. Three of these regimes have been in operation for more than a decade, thus yielding a substantial body of useful data and observational research. With regard to many contested issues, it is no longer necessary to speculate or worry about "sliding down slippery slopes." All four of these regimes have, by now, done various amounts of "sliding," although the assessment of the direction of this movement—down or up those slippery slopes—probably remains a matter of controversy.

Lessons from Four Regimes of Assisted Death

Some fears voiced by critics of PAS and euthanasia have been shown to be unfounded. The number of individuals who take advantage of the possibility of obtaining aid in dying has remained relatively small and for the most part is limited to cases of intractable suffering in terminal illness. As knowledge of the availability of this remedy for inordinate suffering spreads, and the idea of assisted death becomes more acceptable to both doctors and the public, the total number involved increases. Hence the Netherlands, where PAS and euthanasia have been practiced for more than three decades, has the highest percentage of such deaths (Table 6.1).

Concern that assisted death would displace palliative care has likewise been proved groundless. In fact, wherever legislation has been enacted allowing PAS or euthanasia, the provision of palliative care has been increased. In the Netherlands, since the 1990s, palliative care has taken giant steps forward, with palliative care consulting teams being available for both physicians and patients. In Belgium, the legalization of euthanasia was accompanied by passage of a law promoting palliative care. The budget for palliative care was doubled, and by 2007, Belgium ranked third among the European countries in the allocation resources to palliative care. In Oregon, by 2007, 88% of patients dying under provisions of the Death with Dignity Act (DWDA) were under hospice care. Even in Switzerland, where right-to-die organizations have done little if anything to encourage palliative care, various other organizations promoting palliative care have been galvanized into action and have successfully increased their efforts, in response to growing numbers of cases of assisted suicide.

All sides, it appears, want to make sure that patients are not driven to embrace suicide because of inadequate end-of-life care. Increasingly, both advocates of assisted death and supporters of palliative care are moving toward the position that palliative care and assisted death are not mutually exclusive and indeed may complement each other—hastening death may become necessary and acceptable after all other options for alleviating suffering have been carefully explored and exhausted. Both the

TABLE 6.1 Frequency of Assisted Death (Physician-assisted Suicide or Euthanasia) as Percentage of All Deaths

Netherlands (2005)	2.20%
Belgium (2006–2007)	0.44
Switzerland (2001–2002)	0.36
Oregon (2008)	0.19

Canadian Hospice Palliative Care Association and the American Academy of Hospice and Palliative Medicine (AAHPM) have abandoned their earlier principled opposition to PAS and have assumed a position of neutrality on the question of whether PAS should be legalized or remain prohibited. This was done, said a statement issued by the Board of Directors of the AAHPM on February 14, 2007, because "[s]incere, compassionate, morally conscientious individuals stand on either side of this debate."[2]

As we have seen, the Belgian organization Caritas Flanders acknowledges that if a patient persists in his request for euthanasia despite the implementation of the palliative filter procedure, the physician may relieve the patient's suffering through euthanasia. Many patients withdraw their request for assisted death after experiencing the benefits of good palliative care, although for a very small number death becomes agonizing despite the very best efforts to palliate. Moreover, some patients may not want a prolonged death, no matter how well their pain and other serious discomforts (shortness of breath, nausea, vomiting, bed sores) are alleviated. The case of one such patient, "Diane," afflicted with acute myelomonocytic leukemia, who did not wish to linger even in relative comfort, is described by Timothy Quill in a moving article published in 1991.[3]

The rate at which physicians agree to provide assistance in dying gives an indication of how seriously doctors take their role as decision-maker on whether a patient should be helped to die: whether the patient is competent to make the request, whether the patient is in a medically futile condition with unbearable suffering, whether alternative options are available. Available figures show that this rate varies from 37% of granted applications for euthanasia or PAS in the Netherlands in 1995, to 86% in the case of the largest Swiss right-to-die organization, Exit—German Switzerland, in 1996. In many of the cases handled by Exit, the decision is made not by a family doctor but by a physician close to Exit and its philosophy. Moreover, from 2001 to 2004, more than one-third of these applications to Exit involved nonfatal cases, whereas in the Netherlands, over the years, only 9% of those requesting aid in dying have had a life expectancy of more than one month. In Belgium, too, only 7% of those availing themselves of the euthanasia act have been nonterminal patients. The conclusion is inescapable that the practice of Exit—German Switzerland, in line with its philosophy of stressing the autonomy of the person, involves not only assistance in dying but also help in suicide for those who, for various reasons, are tired of life.

The problem of pain control in terminal patients remains to be solved. Despite much progress in end-of-life care, writes one student of the subject, there is still "ample justification for patients to believe that their pain will not be adequately managed."[4] And yet pain, the evidence shows, is usually not the most important reason for seeking assistance in dying. More frequently, it is the desire to be in control of the dying process, fear of loss of dignity, concern about a progressively diminishing quality of life, and not wanting to be a burden. In the context of many European states, where medical care is made available to all irrespective of means, not wanting to be a burden means not wanting to be dependent on the assistance of others for the most elementary aspects of daily living, rather than being a financial liability. The importance of the desire for control is brought out by the fact that many of those who request a lethal medication never use it, and die a natural death. In Oregon, for example, the average rate of such non-use has been 35% during the last ten years.

Oregon, like the rest of the United States, has a far less adequate and universal system of medical care than does Europe. Yet, even here, it has not been the elderly, poor, or uneducated who have sought assistance in dying. As compared with other Oregonians who died from similar diseases, those seeking PAS have been younger, better-educated, and had a higher income. It remains to be seen whether Oregon's experience can be duplicated in other states of the union that have a higher rate of uninsured and underinsured, but it is quite possible that there, too, recourse to assisted death will predominantly involve the better-situated rather than the poor.

A poll conducted by the *Detroit Free Press* found that although 53% of whites in Michigan had an interest in assisted suicide, only 22% of blacks voiced a similar sentiment. Neil Gorsuch, who relates this poll, surmises that this unease on the part of a minority group with large numbers of poor people is due to the inferior medical treatment available to blacks and the fear of being coerced into suicide by the absence of adequate pain relief.[5] In regard to this issue, two long-time students of the problem of assisted death, Timothy Quill and Margaret Battin, have stressed, that although universal access to medical care is indeed urgently needed, it would be highly unfair to those patients who are suffering intolerably despite the availability of excellent palliative care to postpone the option of legal access to physician-assisted death until the problem of universal medical care has been solved. "We do not withhold expensive, marginally effective treatments for the few who might possibly benefit from them because so many lack coverage. Similarly, we do not prevent patients from stopping potentially effective treatment because they may be intentionally seeking to hasten their death or because others might not have access to effective treatment."[6]

If the vulnerable are at risk, conclude Griffiths and his co-authors, "then the place to look for the danger is among the very large number of deaths due to pain relief, palliative/terminal sedation, and abstention from life-prolonging treatment, in many of which the patient or his representative are not involved in the decision-making."[7] This observation about various largely unregulated forms of end-of-life decisions that take place in numbers far exceeding the occurrence of PAS and euthanasia refers to the Netherlands, but it undoubtedly holds true for the rest of the Western world as well. There, too, decisions not to start or to withdraw treatment are common, and are made in full awareness of their life-shortening effect. Terminal sedation is usually accompanied by the withholding of nutrition and hydration which, as one observer puts it, makes it tantamount to "euthanasia, or a kind of 'slow euthanasia.'" The doctrine of the double effect, he adds, may justify sedation but hardly the withholding of food and liquids.[8]

This is not to say that the practice of assisted death in the four regimes examined is free of difficulties and unresolved problems. For example, requests for aid in dying everywhere are required to be voluntary and well-considered. Patients are expected to be competent to make such a request, and yet in the case of patients with a psychiatric disorder that accompanies a severe somatic illness, the capacity for a well-considered request may be impaired. It is well known that the desire for death on the part of very ill patients is often associated with depression, and it is not clear at what point depression precludes rational judgment. At a time when even psychiatrists report finding it difficult to make an accurate diagnosis of depression from a single consultation, can one expect ordinary physicians to distinguish between the depressed mood in a severely ill patient and clinical depression that affects mental competence? Should there be a mandatory "psychiatric filter," even though some psychiatrists question the wisdom of making their profession the final gatekeepers of assisted death? How does one respond to patients who consider a psychiatric examination in their final hours an insufferable indignity?

Another problem involves the scope or reach of a law that allows assistance in suicide. The three European regimes require the presence of lasting and unbearable suffering, whereas Oregon insists that patients be in the terminal phase of their illness. There is a downside to each approach. The criterion of severe suffering could open the door to cases of existential suffering, and involves doctors in the social problem of elderly people who no longer want to live. The insistence that patients be terminal prevents relief for persons with degenerative neurological diseases (such as amyotrophic lateral sclerosis [ALS]), even though their suffering may be pronounced. There is also the dilemma of people with early Alzheimer's disease, who may seek assisted death before the mentally incapacitating disease robs them of the competency to ask for PAS. The Belgian law on euthanasia wisely recognizes the need for special safeguards in cases in which patients are not in a terminal phase of their incurable illness by requiring an examination by a specialist in the disorder and a waiting period of at least one month before the patient's request for assisted death can be acted upon.

Applying the criterion of lasting suffering also raises the dilemma of extremely premature babies, sometimes born with serious disorders or deformities. In such cases, physicians sometimes decide to not initiate or to discontinue treatment. A study of such practices in neonatal clinics in seven European countries published in 2000 revealed that between 61% and 96% of physicians had at least once limited intensive medical measures for such babies.[9] In addition, there arises the question of whether it is ever acceptable deliberately to end the life of newborns and infants who are not dependent on life-sustaining treatment, but whose future quality of life has an extremely poor diagnosis. Who should have final say in such cases to determine what is in the "best interests" of the child? The future livability of severely handicapped newborns, some argue, does not involve a purely medical judgment and introduces an essentially subjective evaluation of quality of life. The decision of parents carries the risk of bias because of the emotional, physical, and financial hardships they face in the long-term care of a severely disabled child. The Groningen Protocol developed in the Netherlands goes a long way toward answering some of these questions, although it has yet to find full acceptance.

Other problems we have noted in the practice of assisted suicide and for which full solutions have yet to be found are the degree of involvement of doctors in the actual suicide, or the difficulty many doctors have in sorting out their motives when they administer large doses of barbiturates to alleviate symptoms. There is also the basic dilemma of devising control procedures and safeguards that, on one hand, will prevent abuses while at the same time will not be excessively intrusive and onerous or undermine the clinical discretion of doctors.

Right-to-die organizations have played an important role in promoting legislation allowing assisted death. Yet, in Switzerland, the strong commitment to patient autonomy has at times also led to a disregard of safeguards designed to prevent abuse. The unseemly haste with which the Swiss organization Dignitas processes large numbers of "suicide tourists" is an extreme case. But, as we have seen, even the more responsible Swiss organization, Exit, because it makes extensive use of physicians who are members of or close to Exit, often appears to act too hastily and does not adequately test the persistence of the death wish. There prevails a right-to-die mentality that has been shown to exert psychological pressure upon vulnerable persons with serious psychological problems. The desire for suicide is often a cry for help, and in some cases there is little indication that alternative options such a palliative care are seriously considered. In the summer of 2009, Canton Zurich and Exit signed an agreement that hopefully will address some of these problems, but other Swiss right-to-die organizations continue to operate in a completely unregulated manner. The Swiss model of assisted death, which slights the role of physicians and often functions in a legal vacuum, is likely to give the idea of assistance in dying a bad name.

A Model Statute for Physician-assisted Suicide

In 1996, nine specialists in the fields of law, medicine, philosophy, and economics proposed a model statute for the regulation of PAS. This model is designed to prevent mistaken decisions, yet provide ready access to relief for patients suffering from terminal illness or unbearable pain.[10] The proposed legislation would legalize PAS but not voluntary euthanasia. The authors stated that restricting the statute to PAS "provides in many cases a stronger assurance of the patient's voluntary resolve to die and of the central role of patient responsibility for the act." The statute's limitation to PAS, they believed, would also bring about a greater acceptance of the model by the public, legislators, and physicians.[11] The proposed legislation is based on American law, but also has wider relevance.

The authors noted that the legal right of patients to decide about life-sustaining treatment, including the right of competent patients to hasten the moment of their death by refusing treatment that would prolong their suffering, has given most patients appropriate control over their own dying. They write:

> However, for some patients who are undergoing severe suffering and confronting an unbearable or meaningless existence, either no life-sustaining treatment is available to be forgone or forgoing such treatment will result in a prolonged, unbearable, and inhumane dying process. Even when optimal care has been given, intolerable distress may remain in these patients, such that they may conclude rationally that hastening death is the only appropriate goal. For these patients, more active means of hastening death are necessary, supported by the very same values that promote patients' well-being and respect their self-determination.[12]

The procedures, conditions, and documentation requirements built into the model statute, the authors stressed, were designed to ensure that PAS "is restricted to patients who are truly terminally ill or suffering from intractable and unbearable illnesses, and whose requests are demonstrably competent, fully informed, voluntary, and enduring." Although these procedures may be viewed as invasive of the privacy of patients and families, they are nevertheless necessary in prevent misuse or abuse of the practice of PAS. They also provide assurance to society that the practice is operating as intended, as well as provide feedback to government and professional bodies about needed refinements and revisions in the practice over time.[13]

In line with these principles, Section 3 of the model statute provides that a licensed physician (the "responsible physician") can provide a

patient with medical means of suicide, provided the following conditions
are met:

1. The patient is eighteen years of age or older.
2. The patient has a terminal illness or an intractable and unbearable
   illness that cannot be cured or successfully palliated and causes
   such severe suffering that a patient prefers death.
3. The patient's request is not the result of a distortion of the patient's
   judgment due to clinical depression or any other mental illness,
   represents the patient's reasoned choice, has been made free of
   undue influence by any person.
4. The request been repeated without self-contradiction on two
   separate occasions at least 14 days apart.

The responsible physician who has provided the means of suicide may
be present and assist the patient at the time that the patient makes use of
such means, as long as the actual use is the knowing, intentional, and voluntary act of the patient.

Section 4 requires the physician, before providing the medical means
of suicide, to:

1. Offer the patient information about all medical care, including
   hospice, that can be made available for the purpose of curing or
   palliating the patient's illness or alleviating symptoms, including
   pain and other discomfort.
2. Offer the patient the opportunity to consult with a social worker or
   similar professional to determine whether services are available that
   could improve the patient's circumstances sufficiently to cause the
   patient to reconsider the request for assistance in suicide.
3. Counsel the patient to inform his family if the physician believes
   that this would be in the patient's interest.
4. Discuss with the patient the means of suicide that can be made
   available and their benefits and burdens. This discussion must be
   witnessed by two adult individuals, at least one of whom is not
   affiliated with any person involved in the care of the patient and
   does not stand to benefit personally from the patient's death.
   The witnesses may question the physician and patient to ascertain

that the patient has indeed heard and understood all of the material information provided by the physician. The physician must document this discussion by means of an audio or video tape or a written summary signed by the patient and the witnesses.

Section 5 and 6 provide that the responsible physician must:

1. Secure a written opinion from a consulting physician who has examined the patient and is qualified to assess that the patient is suffering from a terminal illness or an intractable and unbearable illness.
2. Secure a written opinion from a licensed psychiatrist or other mental health care professional who has examined the patient and is qualified to confirm that the patient's request for assistance in suicide is not the result of distortion of the patient's judgment due to clinical depression or any other mental illness, is reasoned, is fully informed, and is free of undue influence by any person.
3. Place the written opinions described in 1 and 2 in the patient's medical record.
4. Submit a report to the state's regulatory authority, usually the Department of Public Health.

Section 7 allows any individual honestly believing that the requirements of this statute have been met, and if the patient so requests, to be present and assist at the time that the patient makes use of the medical means of suicide, provided that the actual use is the knowing, intentional, and voluntary act of the patient. A licensed pharmacist may dispense the medical means of suicide to a person who presents a valid prescription for such means.

Sections 8, 9, and 10 make the state's regulatory authority responsible for developing the forms of reports to be filed by physicians involved in the assisted suicide. In addition to the place and date of the assisted suicide, the reports are to include the patient's vital statistics and information about insurance. The reports shall not include the name of the patient, but there should be in place an anonymous coding or reference system to enable the regulatory authority or the responsible physician to associate such reports with the patient's medical record. The regulatory authority shall enforce the provisions of the statute and report any violations to the attorney general for criminal prosecution. It shall also report annually to the legislature concerning the operation of the statute. The final sections of the statute deal with issues of confidentiality, conscientious objection, and discrimination that are relatively noncontroversial.

This model act addresses some of the problems that have arisen in the implementation of PAS. In line with European practice, the statute allows PAS not only for patients with a terminal illness but also for those who feel that their suffering is intractable, unbearable, and worse than death. The authors acknowledge that this determination is inherently subjective, but reject a more objective standard as undesirable. Since the statute does not establish a right to PAS, the physician still retains the last word as to whether a particular case warrants relief through assistance in dying. In view of the well-known difficulty general practitioners have in recognizing the presence of depression, the statute requires an evaluation by a psychiatrist or other mental health care professional. There is considerable emphasis on the importance of providing the patient with information on palliative care as a possible alternative to assisted suicide.

The proposed control procedure probably should use the Belgian scheme of putting the physician's report into two envelopes, as a way of safeguarding the privacy of the doctor–patient relationship while at the same time ensuring the possibility of holding offending physicians accountable. Moreover, the control system should function not only as a check on the adherence of doctors to the provisions of the statute but also provide feedback to the medical profession, as occurs in the Netherlands. The public reports of the Dutch review committees contain descriptions of difficult cases, as well as explanations for why the committees decided cases the way they did. In this way, review committees exercise an important educational role and improve the quality of decision-making in the practice of euthanasia.

Other problem areas fare somewhat less well. The model law does not address the issue of severely suffering impaired babies or minors generally. Although the statute requires a written opinion from a second physician, there is no requirement that the consulting physician be fully independent of the responsible physician or that he have special expertise in end-of-life care. The experience of the Netherlands and Belgium has shown that the availability of consultants with extensive knowledge of palliative care can significantly reduce the need for assisted death. Familiarity with palliative care improves the ability of physicians to decide whether the suffering of patients is indeed hopeless. A requirement that the consulting physician be a palliative care expert would create a de facto "palliative filter," as practiced in the facilities run by Caritas Flanders (Belgium). It would also come close to creating a prior review of the decision for assisted death.

Dilemmas and Promise of Legalized Assisted Death

As we have seen, various forms of shortening life are a regular occurrence everywhere, despite the fact that many of these practices violate existing law. We have no hard data for what has been called the "euthanasia underground," but various studies (see Chapter 1) have shown that number to be substantial. The clear advantage of a legal system that allows assisted death is that it provides certain minimum standards of due care, brings these practices out into the open, and makes them subject to legal control. This control, like law enforcement generally, is not perfect. The various control provisions rely on self-reporting, which assumes that most physicians will adhere to prevailing standards of professional integrity. Yet, surely, an imperfect system of control is better than no control at all, which unfortunately is the situation in the currently prevailing euthanasia underground, one characterized by secrecy, deception, inefficiency, and the absence of any kind of protection of the rights and interests of patients.

Although one might expect a greater level of protection from the risk of error and abuse in jurisdictions that directly prohibit the practice of assisted death, two Dutch students of the European scene write that, "the empirical data to date point, perhaps ironically, to the conclusion that the risks of abuse are greater in a climate where euthanasia is prohibited." Prohibition cannot be equated with effective control, and, "conversely, it is equally wrong to assume that the absence of prohibition leads to the uncontrolled or uncontrollable practice of euthanasia. In fact, the available evidence points to the contrary, namely that carefully balanced and measured regulation, which has the support of the medical profession, is far more likely to lead to effective control than outright prohibition which is ignored in practice and attracts widespread cynicism."[14]

In their careful study of the practice of assisted death in Europe, John Griffith and his co-authors come to the same conclusion. Before 2002, Griffiths had been skeptical about the benefits that could be expected from legalizing the practice of euthanasia, but writing ten years later, he concluded that "the available data seem to suggest that legalization of euthanasia leads to less, not more, medical behaviour that potentially shortens life, and to a reduced, not an increased, risk to those particularly vulnerable."[15] In the United States, Margaret Battin has similarly stressed that "legalization and the openness it brings are the best protection against abuse."[16] To put it differently, the "choice we face is not a choice between having no euthanasia and making it legal: rather it is a choice between driving it underground (with all the related concerns about lack of transparency and medical professionalism) and making it visible."[17]

Risks are associated with the legalization of assisted dying, especially in a society like that of the United States. American physicians, unlike Dutch family doctors, usually do not have a long-term close relationship with their patients and have long since abandoned house calls and home care. On the other hand, palliative care and hospice generally function well in the United States, and, if generally available, should make it possible for a regime of assisted death to function effectively as well as sensitively. Supporters of legalizing assisted death therefore rightly insist that such a regime should be instituted only in the context of fully developed end-of-life care. In the words of Timothy Quill, a hospice medical director for eight years:

> Allowing physician-assisted death to be an alternative to good medical care would be immoral and unthinkable. Any intervention that results in a patient's death should be offered only as a last resort, after all reasonable comfort-oriented options have been exhausted. Any proposal considering legitimization of physician-assisted death should require access to comprehensive palliative care as a precondition. The physician providing a second opinion must have extensive experience in caring for the dying. Allowing patients to choose death makes sense only as the final expression of our caring and obligation not to abandon, not as an alternative to the best medical care available.[18]

The absence of legally available assisted dying often encourages violent and inhumane options such as people jumping out of windows or availing themselves of recourse to self-help schemes. Some patients voluntarily stop eating and drinking or ask for and receive terminal sedation. The undesirability of violent suicide and of the spread of the "deathing counterculture" that operates without any kind of professional supervision is obvious, and the other two alternatives to PAS (voluntary fasting and terminal sedation) also have significant downsides. To forego food and drink requires a resolute determination, whereas terminal sedation, not all that different from euthanasia, puts patients into a drug-induced stupor that deprives them of the ability to communicate with family and friends during their final hours.

I am inclined to believe that the prolonged experience with assisted death in the four national entities examined in this study makes it possible to develop a regime that will satisfy the need for dignity in dying, assure accountability, and provide adequate safeguards against abuse. The fact that there are still unresolved issues in all of these regimes does not mean that these issues cannot be successfully addressed. Any such regime should indeed be a work in progress, with its mode of operation carefully studied on a regular basis and revised as problems are detected. The example of the evolving practice of assisted death in the Netherlands, Belgium, and Oregon shows that these are not unrealistic expectations.

APPENDIX 1

THE DUTCH TERMINATION OF LIFE ON REQUEST AND ASSISTED SUICIDE (REVIEW PROCEDURES) ACT[*]

Amended legislative proposal

28 November 2000

We BEATRIX, by the grace of God, Queen of the Netherlands, Princess of Orange-Nassau, etc., etc. etc.

Greetings to all who shall see or hear these presents! Be it known:

Whereas We have considered that it is desired to include a ground for exemption from criminal liability for the physician who with due observance of the requirements of due care to be laid down by law terminates a life on request or assists in a suicide of another person, and to provide a statutory notification and review procedure;

We, therefore, having heard the Council of State, and in consultation with the States General, have approved and decreed as We hereby approve and decree:

Chapter I. Definitions of Terms

Article 1

For the purposes of this Act:

   a. Our Ministers mean the Ministers of Justice and of Health, Welfare and Sports;

---

[*] Official translation provided by the Dutch Departments of Justice and Foreign Affairs, to be found at *http://www.justitie.nl* and *http://www.minbuza.nl.*

b. assisted suicide means intentionally assisting in a suicide of another person or procuring for that other person the means referred to in Article 294 second paragraph second sentence of the Penal Code;

c. the physician means the physician who according to the notification has terminated a life on request or assisted in a suicide;

d. the consultant means the physician who has been consulted with respect to the intention by the physician to terminate a life on request or to assist in a suicide;

e. the providers of care mean the providers of care referred to in Article 446 first paragraph of Book 7 of the Civil Code (*Burgerlijk Wetboek*);

f. the committee means a regional review committee referred to in Article 3;

g. the regional inspector means the regional inspector of the Health Care Inspectorate of the Public Health Supervisory Service.

Chapter II. Requirements of Due Care

Article 2

1. The requirements of due care, referred to in Article 293 second paragraph Penal Code mean that the physician:

   a. holds the conviction that the request by the patient was voluntary and well-considered,

   b. holds the conviction that the patient's suffering was lasting and unbearable,

   c. has informed the patient about the situation he was in and about his prospects,

   d. and the patient hold the conviction that there was no other reasonable solution for the situation he was in,

   e. has consulted at least one other, independent physician who has seen the patient and has given his written opinion on the requirements of due care, referred to in parts a—d, and

   f. has terminated a life or assisted in a suicide with due care.

2. If the patient aged sixteen years or older is no longer capable of expressing his will, but prior to reaching this condition was deemed to have a reasonable understanding of his interests and has made a written statement containing a request for termination of life, the physician may carry out this request. The requirements of due care, referred to in the first paragraph, apply *mutatis mutandis*.

3. If the minor patient has attained an age between sixteen and eighteen years and may be deemed to have a reasonable understanding of his interests, the physician may carry out the patient's request for termination of life or assisted suicide, after the parent or the parents exercising parental authority and/or his guardian have been involved in the decision process.

4. If the minor patient is aged between twelve and sixteen years and may be deemed to have a reasonable understanding of his interests, the physician may carry out the patient's request, provided always that the parent or the parents exercising parental authority and/or his guardian agree with the termination of life or the assisted suicide. The second paragraph applies *mutatis mutandis.*

Chapter III. The Regional Review Committees for Termination of Life on Request and Assisted Suicide

Paragraph 1: Establishment, composition and appointment

Article 3

1. There are regional committees for the review of notifications of cases of termination of life on request and assistance in a suicide as referred to in Article 293 second paragraph or 294 second paragraph second sentence, respectively, of the Penal Code.

2. A committee is composed of an uneven number of members, including at any rate one legal specialist, also chairman, one physician and one expert on ethical or philosophical issues

3. The committee also contains deputy members of each of the categories listed in the first sentence.

Article 4

1. The chairman and the members, as well as the deputy members are appointed by Our Ministers for a period of six years. They may be re-appointed one time for another period of six years.

2. A committee has a secretary and one or more deputy secretaries, all legal specialists, appointed by Our Ministers. The secretary has an advisory role in the committee meetings.

3. The secretary may solely be held accountable by the committee for his activities for the committee.

Paragraph 2: Dismissal

Article 5

Our Ministers may at any time dismiss the chairman and the members, as well as the deputy members at their own request.

Article 6

Our Ministers may dismiss the chairman and the members, as well as the deputy members for reasons of unsuitability or incompetence or for other important reasons.

Paragraph 3: Remuneration

Article 7

The chairman and the members, as well as the deputy members receive a holiday allowance as well as a reimbursement of the travel and accommodation expenses according to the existing government scheme insofar as these expenses are not otherwise reimbursed from the State Funds.

Paragraph 4: Duties and powers

Articles 8

1. The committee assesses on the basis of the report referred to in Article 7 second paragraph of the Burial and Cremation Act whether the physician who has terminated a life on request or assisted in a suicide has acted in accordance with the requirements of due care, referred to in Article 2.
2. The committee may request the physician to supplement his report in writing or verbally, where this is necessary for a proper assessment of the physician's actions.
3. The committee may make enquiries at the municipal autopsist, the consultant or the providers of care involved where this is necessary for a proper assessment of the physician's actions.

Article 9

1. The committee informs the physician within six weeks of the receipt of the report referred to in Article 8 first paragraph in writing of its motivated opinion.
2. The committee informs the Board of Procurators General and the regional health care inspector of its opinion:
   a. if the committee is of the opinion that the physician has failed to act in accordance with the requirements of due care, referred to in Article 2; or
   b. if a situation occurs as referred to in Article 12, final sentence of the Burial and Cremation Act.

   The committee shall inform the physician of this.
3. The term referred to in the first paragraph may be extended one time by a maximum period of six weeks. The committee shall inform the physician of this.
4. The committee may provide a further, verbal explanation on its opinion to the physician. This verbal explanation may take place at the request of the committee or at the request of the physician.

Article 10

The committee is obliged to provide all information to the public prosecutor, at his request, which he may need:

1.° for the benefit of the assessment of the physician's actions in the case referred to in Article 9 second paragraph; or
2.° for the benefit of a criminal investigation.

The committee shall inform the physician of any provision of information to the public prosecutor.

Paragraph 6: Working method

Article 11

The committee shall ensure the registration of the cases of termination of life or assisted suicide reported for assessment. Further rules on this may be laid down by a ministerial regulation by Our Ministers.

Article 12

1. An opinion is adopted by a simple majority of votes.
2. An opinion may only be adopted by the committee provided all committee members have participated in the vote.

Article 13

At least twice a year, the chairmen of the regional review committees conduct consultations with one another with respect to the working method and the performance of the committees. A representative of the Board of Procurators General and a representative of the Health Care Inspectorate of the Public Health Supervisory Service are invited to attend these consultations.

Paragraph 7: Secrecy and exemption

Article 14

The members and deputy members of the committee are under an obligation of secrecy to keep confidential any information acquired in the performance of their duties, except where any statutory regulation obliges them to divulge this information or where the necessity to divulge information ensues from their duties.

Article 15

A member of the committee that serves on the committee in the treatment of a case exempts himself and may be challenged if there are facts or circumstances that may affect the impartiality of his opinion.

Article 16

A member, a deputy member and the secretary of the committee refrain from rendering an opinion on the intention by a physician to terminate a life on request or to assist in a suicide.

Paragraph 8: Report

Article 17

1. Not later than 1 April, the committees issue a joint annual report to Our Ministers on the activities of the past calendar year. Our Ministers shall lay down a model for this by means of a ministerial regulation.
2. The report on the activities referred to in the first paragraph shall at any rate include the following:
   a. the number of reported cases of termination of life on request and assisted suicide on which the committee has rendered an opinion;
   b. the nature of these cases;
   c. the opinions and the considerations involved.

Article 18

Annually, at the occasion of the submission of the budget to the States General, Our Ministers shall issue a report with respect to the performance of the committees further to the report on the activities as referred to in Article 17 first paragraph.

Article 19

1. On the recommendation of Our Ministers, rules shall be laid down by order in council regarding the committees with respect to
   a. their number and their territorial jurisdiction;
   b. their domicile.
2. Our Ministers may lay down further rules by or pursuant to an order in council regarding the committees with respect to
   a. their size and composition;
   b. their working method and reports.

Chapter IV. Amendments to other Acts

Article 20

The Penal Code shall be amended as follows:

A.

Article 293 shall read:

Article 293

1. A person who terminates the life of another person at that other person's express and earnest request is liable to a term of imprisonment of not more than twelve years or a fine of the fifth category.
2. The offence referred to in the first paragraph shall not be punishable if it has been committed by a physician who has met the requirements of due care as referred to in Article 2 of the Termination of Life on Request and Assisted Suicide (Review Procedures) Act and who informs the municipal autopsist of this in accordance with Article 7 second paragraph of the Burial and Cremation Act.

B.

Article 294 shall read:

Article 294

1. A person who intentionally incites another to commit suicide, is liable to a term of imprisonment of not more than three years or a fine of the fourth category, where the suicide ensues.
2. A person who intentionally assists in the suicide of another or procures for that other person the means to commit suicide, is liable to a term of imprisonment of not more than three years or a fine of the fourth category, where the suicide ensues. Article 293 second paragraph applies *mutatis mutandis.*

C. In Article 295, the following is inserted after '293': first paragraph.

D. In Article 422, the following is inserted after '293': first paragraph.

Article 21

The Burial and Cremation Act shall be amended as follows:

A.

Article 7 shall read:

Article 7

1. A person who has performed a postmortem shall issue a death certificate if he is convinced that death has occurred as a result of a natural cause.
2. If the death was the result of the application of termination of life on request or assisted suicide as referred to in Article 293 second paragraph or Article 294 second paragraph second sentence, respectively, of the Penal Code, the attending physician shall not issue a death certificate and shall promptly notify the municipal autopsist or one of the municipal autopsists of the cause of death by completing a form. The physician shall supplement this form with a reasoned report with respect to the due observance of the requirements of due care referred to in Article 2 of the Termination of Life on Request and Assisted Suicide (Review Procedures) act.
3. If the attending physician in other cases than referred to in the second paragraph believes that he may not issue a death certificate, he must promptly notify the municipal autopsist or one of the municipal autopsists of this by completing a form.

B.

Article 9 shall read:

Article 9

1. The form and the set-up of the models of the death certificate to be issued by the attending physician and by the municipal autopsist shall be laid down by order in council.
2. The form and the set-up of the models of the notification and the report referred to in Article 7 second paragraph, of the notification referred to in Article 7 third paragraph and of the forms referred to in Article 10 first and second paragraph shall be laid down by order in council on the

recommendation of Our Minister of Justice and Our Minister of Health, Welfare and Sports.

C.

Article 10 shall read:

Article 10

1. If the municipal autopsist is of the opinion that he cannot issue a death certificate, he shall promptly report this to the public prosecutor by completing a form and he shall promptly notify the registrar of births, deaths and marriages.
2. In the event of a notification as referred to in Article 7 second paragraph and without prejudice to the first paragraph, the municipal autopsist shall promptly report to the regional review committee referred to in Article 3 of the Termination of Life on Request and Assisted Suicide (Review Procedures) Act by completing a form. He shall enclose a reasoned report as referred to in Article 7 second paragraph.

D.

The following sentence shall be added to Article 12, reading: If the public prosecutor, in the cases referred to in Article 7 second paragraph, is of the opinion that he cannot issue a certificate of no objection against the burial or cremation, he shall promptly inform the municipal autopsist and the regional review committee referred to in Article 3 of the Termination of Life on Request and Assisted Suicide (Review Procedures) Act of this.

E.

In Article 81, first part, '7, first paragraph' shall be replaced by '7, first and second paragraph'.

Article 22

The General Administrative Law Act (*Algemene wet bestuursrecht*) shall be amended as follows: At the end of part d of Article 1:6, the full stop shall be replaced by a semicolon and the following shall be added to the fifth part, reading:

e. decisions and actions in the implementation of the Termination of Life and Assisted Suicide (Review Procedures) Act.

Chapter V. Final Provisions

Article 23

This Act shall take effect as of a date to be determined by Royal Decree.

Article 24

This Act may be cited as: Termination of Life on Request and Assisted Suicide (Review Procedures) Act.

We hereby order and command that this Act shall be published in the *Bulletin of Acts and Decrees* and that all ministerial departments, authorities, bodies and officials whom it may concern shall diligently implement it.

Done

The Minister of Justice,

The Minister of Health, Welfare and Sports.

Upper House, parliamentary year 2000-2001, 26 691, no 137

APPENDIX 2

THE BELGIAN ACT ON EUTHANASIA OF 28 MAY 2002[*]

ALBERT II, King of the Belgians,
To all those present now and in the future, greetings.
The Chambers have approved and We sanction what follows:

Section 1

This law governs a matter provided in article 78 of the Constitution.

Chapter I: General provisions

Section 2

For the purposes of this Act, euthanasia is defined as intentionally terminating life by someone other than the person concerned, at the latter's request.

Chapter II: Conditions and procedure

Section 3

§1. The physician who performs euthanasia commits no criminal offence when he/she ensures that:
  – the patient has attained the age of majority or is an emancipated minor, and is legally competent and conscious at the moment of making the request;

---

[*] Translation provided by Dale Kidd (European Centre for Ethics, Catholic University of Leuven) under the scientific supervision of Prof, Herman Nys, Centre for Biomedical Ethics and Law, Faculty of Medicine, Catholic University of Leuven (Belgium).

- the request is voluntary, well-considered and repeated, and is not the result of any external pressure;
- the patient is in a medically futile condition of constant and unbearable physical or mental suffering that can not be alleviated, resulting from a serious and incurable disorder caused by illness or accident;

and when he/she has respected the conditions and procedures as provided in this Act.

§2. Without prejudice to any additional conditions imposed by the physician on his/her own action, before carrying out euthanasia he/she must in each case:

1) inform the patient about his/her health condition and life expectancy, discuss with the patient his/her request for euthanasia and the possible therapeutic and palliative courses of action and their consequences. Together with the patient, the physician must come to the belief that there is no reasonable alternative to the patient's situation and that the patient's request is completely voluntary;

2) be certain of the patient's constant physical or mental suffering and of the durable nature of his/her request. To this end, the physician has several conversations with the patient spread out over a reasonable period of time, taking into account the progress of the patient's condition;

3) consult another physician about the serious and incurable character of the disorder and inform him/her about the reasons for this consultation. The physician consulted reviews the medical record, examines the patient and must be certain of the patient's constant and unbearable physical or mental suffering that cannot be alleviated. The physician consulted reports on his/her findings.

The physician consulted must be independent of the patient as well as of the attending physician and must be competent to give an opinion about the disorder in question. The attending physician informs the patient about the results of this consultation;

4) if there is a nursing team that has regular contact with the patient; discuss the request of the patient with the nursing team or its members,

5) if the patient so desires, discuss his/her request with relatives appointed by the patient;

6) be certain that the patient has had the opportunity to discuss his/her request with the persons that he/she wanted to meet.

§3. If the physician believes the patient is dearly not expected to die in the near future, he/she must also:

1) consult a second physician, who is a psychiatrist or a specialist in the disorder in question, and inform him/her of the reasons for such a consultation. The physician consulted reviews the medical record, examines the patient and must ensure himself about the constant and unbearable physical or mental suffering that cannot be alleviated, and of the- voluntary, well-considered and repeated character of the euthanasia request. The physician consulted reports on his/her findings. The physician consulted must be independent of the patient as well as of the physician initially consulted. The physician informs the patient about the results of this consultation;

2) allow at least one month between the patient's written request and the act of euthanasia.

§4. The patient's request must be in writing. The document is drawn up, dated and signed by the patient himself/herself. If the patient is not capable of doing this, the document is drawn up by a person designated by the patient. This person must have attained the age of majority and must not have any material interest in the death of the patient.

This person indicates that the patient is incapable of formulating his/her request in writing and the reasons why. In such a case the request is drafted in the presence of the physician whose name is mentioned on the document. This document must be annexed to the medical record.

The patient may revoke his/her request at any time, in which case the document is removed from the medical record and returned to the patient.

§5. All the requests formulated by the patient, as well as any actions by the attending physician and their results, including the report(s) of the consulted physician(s), are regularly noted in the patient's medical record.

Chapter III: The advance directive

Section 4

§1. In cases where one is no longer able to express one's will, every legally competent person of age, or emancipated minor, can draw up an advance

directive instructing a physician to perform euthanasia if the physician ensures that:
– the patient suffers from a serious and incurable disorder, caused by illness or accident;
– the patient is no longer conscious;
– this condition is irreversible given the current state of medical science.

In the advance directive, one or more person(s) taken in confidence can be designated in order of preference, who inform(s) the attending physician about the patient's will. Each person taken in confidence replaces his or her predecessor as mentioned in the advance directive, in the case of refusal, hindrance, incompetence or death. The patient's attending physician, the physician consulted and the members of the nursing team may not act as persons taken in confidence.

The advance directive may be drafted at any moment. It must be composed in writing in the presence of two witnesses, at least one of whom has no material interest in the death of the patient and it must be dated and signed by the drafter, the witnesses and by the person(s) taken in confidence, if applicable.

If a person who wishes to draft an advance directive is permanently physically incapable of writing and signing an advance directive, he/she may designate a person who is of age, and who has no material interest in the death of the person in question, to draft the request in writing, in the presence of two witnesses who have attained the age of majority and at least one of whom has no material interest in the patient's death. The advance directive indicates that the person in question is incapable of signing and why. The advance directive must be dated and signed by the drafter, by the witnesses and by the person(s) taken in confidence, if applicable.

A medical certificate must be annexed to the advance directive proving that the person in question is permanently physically incapable of drafting and signing the advance directive.

An advance directive is only valid if it is drafted or confirmed no more than five years prior to the person's loss of the ability to express his/her wishes.

The advance directive may be amended or revoked at any time.

The King determines the manner in which the advance directive is drafted, registered and confirmed or revoked, and the manner in which it is communicated to the physicians involved via the offices of the National Register.

§2. The physician who performs euthanasia, in consequence of an advance directive as referred to in §1, commits no criminal offence when he ensures that:

- the patient suffers from a serious and incurable disorder, caused by illness or accident;
- the patient is unconscious;
- and this condition is irreversible given the current state of medical science;

and when he/she has respected the conditions and procedures as provided in this Act.

Without prejudice to any additional conditions imposed by the physician on his/her own action, before carrying out euthanasia he/she must:

1) consult another physician about the irreversibility of the patient's medical condition and inform him/her about the reasons for this consultation. The physician consulted consults the medical record and examines the patient. He/she reports on his/her findings.

   When the advance directive names a person taken in confidence, the latter will be informed about the results of this consultation by the attending physician.

   The physician consulted must be independent of the patient as well as of the attending physician and must be competent to give an opinion about the disorder in question;

2) if there is a nursing team that has regular contact with the patient, discuss the content of the advance directive with that team or its members;

3) if a person taken in confidence is designated in the advance directive, discuss the request with that person;

4) if a person taken in confidence is designated in the advance directive, discuss the content of the advance directive with the relatives of the patient designated by the person taken in confidence.

The advance directive, as well as all actions by the attending physician and their results, including the report of the consulted physician, are regularly noted in the patient's medical record.

Chapter IV: Notification

Section 5

Any physician who has performed euthanasia is required to fill in a registration form, drawn up by the Federal Control and Evaluation Commission established by section 6 of this Act, and to deliver this document to the Commission within four working days.

Chapter V: The Federal Control and Evaluation Commission

Section 6

§1. For the implementation of this Act, a Federal Control and Evaluation Commission is established, hereafter referred to as "the commission".

§2. The commission is composed of sixteen members, appointed on the basis of their knowledge and experience in the issues belonging to the commission's jurisdiction. Eight members are doctors of medicine, of whom at least four are professors at a university in Belgium. Four members are professors of law at a university in Belgium, or practising lawyers. Four members are drawn from groups that deal with the problem of incurably ill patients. Membership in the commission cannot be combined with a post in one of the legislative bodies or with a post as a member of the federal government or one of the regional or community governments.

While respecting language parity—where each linguistic group has at least three candidates of each sex—and ensuring pluralistic representation, the members of the commission are appointed by royal decree enacted after deliberation in the Council of Ministers for a four-year term, which may be extended, from a double list of candidates put forward by the Senate, A member's mandate is terminated *de jure* if the member loses the capacity on the basis of which he/she is appointed. The candidates not appointed as sitting members are appointed as substitutes, in the order determined by a list. The commission is chaired by a Dutch-speaking and a French-speaking member. These chairpersons are elected by the commission members of the respective linguistic group.

The commission's decisions are only valid if there is a quorum present of two-thirds of the members.

§3. The commission establishes its own internal regulations.

Section 7

The commission drafts a registration form that must be filled in by the physician whenever he/she performs euthanasia. This document consists of two parts. The first part must be placed under seal by the physician. It includes the following information:

1) the patient's full name and address;
2) the full name, address and health insurance institute registration number of the attending physician;
3) the full name, address and health insurance institute registration number of the physician(s) consulted about the euthanasia request;
4) the full name, address and capacity of all persons consulted by the attending physician, and the date of these consultations;
5) if there exists an advance directive in which one or more persons taken in confidence are designated, the full name of such person(s).

The document's first part is confidential, and is supplied to the commission by the physician. It can only be consulted following a decision by the commission. Under no circumstances the commission may use this document for its evaluation.

The second part is also confidential. It includes the following information:

1) the patient's sex, date of birth and place of birth;
2) the date, time and place of death;
3) the nature of the serious and incurable condition, caused by accident or illness, from which the patient suffered;
4) the nature of the constant and unbearable suffering;
5) the reasons why this suffering could not be alleviated;
6) the elements underlying the assurance that the request is voluntary, well-considered and repeated, and not the result of any external pressure;
7) whether one can expect that the patient would die within the foreseeable future;
8) whether an advance directive has been drafted;
9) the procedure followed by the physician;
10) the capacity of the physician(s) consulted, the recommendations and the information from these consultations;
11) the capacity of the persons consulted by the physician, and the date of these consultations;
12) the manner in which euthanasia was performed and the pharmaceuticals used.

Section 8

The commission studies the completed registration form submitted to it by the attending physician. On the basis of the second part of the registration form, the commission determines whether the euthanasia was performed in accordance with the conditions and the procedure stipulated in this Act. In cases of doubt, the commission may decide by simple majority to revoke anonymity and examine the first part of the registration form. The commission may request the attending physician to provide any information from the medical record having to do with the euthanasia.

The commission hands down a verdict within two months.

If, in a decision taken with a two-thirds majority, the commission is of the opinion that the conditions laid down in this Act have not been fulfilled, then it turns the case over to the public prosecutor of the jurisdiction in which the patient died.

If, after anonymity has been revoked, facts or circumstances come to light which would compromise the independence or impartiality of one of the commission members, this member will have an opportunity to explain or to be challenged during the discussion of this matter in the commission.

Section 9

For the benefit of the legislative chambers, the commission will draft the following reports, the first time within two years of this Act's coming into force and every two years thereafter:

a) a statistical report processing the information from the second part of the completed registration forms submitted by physicians pursuant to section 8;
b) a report in which the implementation of the law is indicated and evaluated;
c) if required, recommendations that could lead to new legislation or other measures concerning the execution of this Act.

For the purpose of carrying out this task, the commission may seek additional information from the various public services and institutions. The information thus gathered is confidential. None of these documents may reveal the identities of any persons named in the dossiers submitted to the commission for the purposes of the review as determined in section 8.

The commission can decide to supply statistical and purely technical data, purged of any personal information, to university research teams that submit a reasoned request for such data.

The commission can grant hearings to experts.

Section 10

The King places an administration at the commission's disposal in order to carry out its legal functions. The composition and language framework of the administrative personnel are established by royal decree, following consultation in the Council of Ministers, on the recommendation of the Minister of Health and the Minister of Justice.

Section 11

The commission's operating costs and personnel costs, including remuneration for its members, are divided equally between the budget of the Minister of Health and the budget of the Minister of Justice.

Section 12

Any person who is involved, in whatever capacity, in implementing this Act is required to maintain confidentiality regarding the information provided to him/her in the exercise of his/her function. He/she is subject to section 458 of the Penal Code.

Section 13

Within six months of submitting the first report and the commission's recommendations referred to in section 9, if any, a debate is to be held in the Chambers of Parliament. The six-month period is suspended during the time that Parliament is dissolved and/or during the time there is no government having the confidence of Parliament.

Chapter VI: Special Provisions

Section 14

The request and the advance directive referred to in sections 3 and 4 of this Act are not compulsory in nature.

No physician may be compelled to perform euthanasia.

No other person may be compelled to assist in performing euthanasia.

Should the physician consulted refuse to perform euthanasia, then he/she must inform the patient and the persons taken in confidence, if any, of this fact in a timely manner, and explain his/her reasons for such refusal. If the refusal is based on medical reasons, then these reasons are noted in the patient's medical record.

At the request of the patient or the person taken in confidence, the physician who refuses to perform euthanasia must communicate the patient's medical record to the physician designated by the patient or person taken in confidence.

Section 15

Any person who dies as a result of euthanasia performed in accordance with the conditions established by this Act is deemed to have died of natural causes for the purposes of contracts he/she had entered into, in particular insurance contracts.

The provisions of section 909 of the Civil Code apply to the members of the nursing team referred to in section 3 of this Act.

Section 16

This Act comes into force no later than three months following publication in the *Official Belgian Gazette*.

Promulgate the present Act, order that it be sealed with the seal of the State and published in the *Official Belgian Gazette*.

Issued at Brussels, 28th May 2002.

ALBERT

for the King:
the Minister of Justice,
M. VERWILGHEN
sealed with the seal of the State:
the Minister of Justice,
M. VERWILGHEN

APPENDIX 3

SWISS CRIMINAL CODE OF 1937 (AS OF OCTOBER 1, 2008)

Art. 114

Wer aus achtenswerten Beweggründen, namentlich aus Mitleid, einen Menschen auf dessen ernsthaftes und eindringliches Verlangen tötet, wird mit Freiheitsstrafe bis zu drei Jahren oder Geldstrafe bestraft.

Art. 115

Wer aus selbstsüchtigen Beweggründen jemanden zum Selbstmorde verleitet oder ihm dazu Hilfe leistet, wird, wenn der Selbstmord ausgeführt oder versucht wurde, mit Freiheitsstrafe bis zu fünf Jahren oder Geldstrafe bestraft.

APPENDIX 4

THE OREGON DEATH WITH DIGNITY ACT
OREGON REVISED STATUTES

(General Provisions)

(Section 1)

Note: The division headings, subdivision headings and leadlines for 127.800 to 127.890, 127.895 and 127.897 were enacted as part of Ballot Measure 16 (1994) and were not provided by Legislative Counsel.

127.800 §1.01. Definitions. The following words and phrases, whenever used in ORS 127.800 to 127.897, have the following meanings:

(1) "Adult" means an individual who is 18 years of age or older.

(2) "Attending physician" means the physician who has primary responsibility for the care of the patient and treatment of the patient's terminal disease.

(3) "Capable" means that in the opinion of a court or in the opinion of the patient's attending physician or consulting physician, psychiatrist or psychologist, a patient has the ability to make and communicate health care decisions to health care providers, including communication through persons familiar with the patient's manner of communicating if those persons are available.

(4) "Consulting physician" means a physician who is qualified by specialty or experience to make a professional diagnosis and prognosis regarding the patient's disease.

(5) "Counseling" means one or more consultations as necessary between a state licensed psychiatrist or psychologist and a patient for the purpose of determining that the patient is capable and not suffering from a psychiatric or psychological disorder or depression causing impaired judgment.

(6) "Health care provider" means a person licensed, certified or otherwise authorized or permitted by the law of this state to administer health care or dispense medication in the ordinary course of business or practice of a profession, and includes a health care facility.

(7) "Informed decision" means a decision by a qualified patient, to request and obtain a prescription to end his or her life in a humane and dignified manner, that is based on an appreciation of the relevant facts and after being fully informed by the attending physician of:

(a) His or her medical diagnosis;

(b) His or her prognosis;

(c) The potential risks associated with taking the medication to be prescribed;

(d) The probable result of taking the medication to be prescribed; and

(e) The feasible alternatives, including, but not limited to, comfort care, hospice care and pain control.

(8) "Medically confirmed" means the medical opinion of the attending physician has been confirmed by a consulting physician who has examined the patient and the patient's relevant medical records.

(9) "Patient" means a person who is under the care of a physician.

(10) "Physician" means a doctor of medicine or osteopathy licensed to practice medicine by the Board of Medical Examiners for the State of Oregon.

(11) "Qualified patient" means a capable adult who is a resident of Oregon and has satisfied the requirements of ORS 127.800 to 127.897 in order to obtain a prescription for medication to end his or her life in a humane and dignified manner.

(12) "Terminal disease" means an incurable and irreversible disease that has been medically confirmed and will, within reasonable medical judgment, produce death within six months. [1995 c.3 §1.01; 1999 c.423 §1]

(Written Request for Medication to End One's Life in a Humane and Dignified Manner)

(Section 2)

127.805 §2.01. Who may initiate a written request for medication. (1) An adult who is capable, is a resident of Oregon, and has been determined by the attending physician and consulting physician to be suffering from a terminal disease, and who has voluntarily expressed his or her wish to die, may make a written request for medication for the purpose of ending his or her life in a humane and dignified manner in accordance with ORS 127.800 to 127.897.

(2) No person shall qualify under the provisions of ORS 127.800 to 127.897 solely because of age or disability. [1995 c.3 §2.01; 1999 c.423 §2]

127.810 §2.02. Form of the written request. (1) A valid request for medication under ORS 127.800 to 127.897 shall be in substantially the form described in ORS 127.897, signed and dated by the patient and witnessed by at least two individuals who, in the presence of the patient, attest that to the best of their knowledge and belief the patient is capable, acting voluntarily, and is not being coerced to sign the request.

(2) One of the witnesses shall be a person who is not:
    (a) A relative of the patient by blood, marriage or adoption;
    (b) A person who at the time the request is signed would be entitled to any portion of the estate of the qualified patient upon death under any will or by operation of law; or
    (c) An owner, operator or employee of a health care facility where the qualified patient is receiving medical treatment or is a resident.
(3) The patient's attending physician at the time the request is signed shall not be a witness.
(4) If the patient is a patient in a long term care facility at the time the written request is made, one of the witnesses shall be an individual designated by the facility and having the qualifications specified by the Department of Human Services by rule. [1995 c.3 §2.02]

(Safeguards)

(Section 3)

127.815 §3.01. Attending physician responsibilities. (1) The attending physician shall:

    (a) Make the initial determination of whether a patient has a terminal disease, is capable, and has made the request voluntarily;
    (b) Request that the patient demonstrate Oregon residency pursuant to ORS 127.860;
    (c) To ensure that the patient is making an informed decision, inform the patient of:
        (A) His or her medical diagnosis;
        (B) His or her prognosis;
        (C) The potential risks associated with taking the medication to be prescribed;
        (D) The probable result of taking the medication to be prescribed; and
        (E) The feasible alternatives, including, but not limited to, comfort care, hospice care and pain control;

(d) Refer the patient to a consulting physician for medical confirmation of the diagnosis, and for a determination that the patient is capable and acting voluntarily;

(e) Refer the patient for counseling if appropriate pursuant to ORS 127.825;

(f) Recommend that the patient notify next of kin;

(g) Counsel the patient about the importance of having another person present when the patient takes the medication prescribed pursuant to ORS 127.800 to 127.897 and of not taking the medication in a public place;

(h) Inform the patient that he or she has an opportunity to rescind the request at any time and in any manner, and offer the patient an opportunity to rescind at the end of the 15 day waiting period pursuant to ORS 127.840;

(i) Verify, immediately prior to writing the prescription for medication under ORS 127.800 to 127.897, that the patient is making an informed decision;

(j) Fulfill the medical record documentation requirements of ORS 127.855;

(k) Ensure that all appropriate steps are carried out in accordance with ORS 127.800 to 127.897 prior to writing a prescription for medication to enable a qualified patient to end his or her life in a humane and dignified manner; and

(L) (A)Dispense medications directly, including ancillary medications intended to facilitate the desired effect to minimize the patient's discomfort, provided the attending physician is registered as a dispensing physician with the Board of Medical Examiners, has a current Drug Enforcement Administration certificate and complies with any applicable administrative rule; or

(B) With the patient's written consent:

(i) Contact a pharmacist and inform the pharmacist of the prescription; and

(ii) Deliver the written prescription personally or by mail to the pharmacist, who will dispense the medications to either the patient, the attending physician or an expressly identified agent of the patient.

(2) Notwithstanding any other provision of law, the attending physician may sign the patient's death certificate. [1995 c.3 §3.01; 1999 c.423 §3]

127.820 §3.02. Consulting physician confirmation. Before a patient is qualified under ORS 127.800 to 127.897, a consulting physician shall examine the patient and his or her relevant medical records and confirm, in writing, the attending physician's diagnosis that the patient is suffering from a terminal disease, and verify that the patient is capable, is acting voluntarily and has made an informed decision. [1995 c.3 §3.02]

127.825 §3.03. Counseling referral. If in the opinion of the attending physician or the consulting physician a patient may be suffering from a psychiatric or psychological disorder or depression causing impaired judgment, either physician shall refer the patient for counseling. No medication to end a patient's life in a humane and dignified manner shall be prescribed until the person performing the counseling determines that the patient is not suffering from a psychiatric or psychological disorder or depression causing impaired judgment. [1995 c.3 §3.03; 1999 c.423 §4]

127.830 §3.04. Informed decision. No person shall receive a prescription for medication to end his or her life in a humane and dignified manner unless he or she has made an informed decision as defined in ORS 127.800 (7). Immediately prior to writing a prescription for medication under ORS 127.800 to 127.897, the attending physician shall verify that the patient is making an informed decision. [1995 c.3 §3.04]

127.835 §3.05. Family notification. The attending physician shall recommend that the patient notify the next of kin of his or her request for medication pursuant to ORS 127.800 to 127.897. A patient who declines or is unable to notify next of kin shall not have his or her request denied for that reason. [1995 c.3 §3.05; 1999 c.423 §6]

127.840 §3.06. Written and oral requests. In order to receive a prescription for medication to end his or her life in a humane and dignified manner, a qualified patient shall have made an oral request and a written request, and reiterate the oral request to his or her attending physician no less than fifteen (15) days after making the initial oral request. At the time the qualified patient makes his or her second oral request, the attending physician shall offer the patient an opportunity to rescind the request. [1995 c.3 §3.06]

127.845 §3.07. Right to rescind request. A patient may rescind his or her request at any time and in any manner without regard to his or her mental state. No prescription for medication under ORS 127.800 to 127.897 may be written without the attending physician offering the qualified patient an opportunity to rescind the request. [1995 c.3 §3.07]

127.850 §3.08. Waiting periods. No less than fifteen (15) days shall elapse between the patient's initial oral request and the writing of a prescription under ORS

127.800 to 127.897. No less than 48 hours shall elapse between the patient's written request and the writing of a prescription under ORS 127.800 to 127.897. [1995 c.3 §3.08]

127.855 §3.09. Medical record documentation requirements. The following shall be documented or filed in the patient's medical record:

1) All oral requests by a patient for medication to end his or her life in a humane and dignified manner;

2) All written requests by a patient for medication to end his or her life in a humane and dignified manner;

3) The attending physician's diagnosis and prognosis, determination that the patient is capable, acting voluntarily and has made an informed decision;

4) The consulting physician's diagnosis and prognosis, and verification that the patient is capable, acting voluntarily and has made an informed decision;

5) A report of the outcome and determinations made during counseling, if performed;

6) The attending physician's offer to the patient to rescind his or her request at the time of the patient's second oral request pursuant to ORS 127.840; and

7) A note by the attending physician indicating that all requirements under ORS 127.800 to 127.897 have been met and indicating the steps taken to carry out the request, including a notation of the medication prescribed. [1995 c.3 §3.09]

127.860 §3.10. Residency requirement. Only requests made by Oregon residents under ORS 127.800 to 127.897 shall be granted. Factors demonstrating Oregon residency include but are not limited to:

(1) Possession of an Oregon driver license;

(2) Registration to vote in Oregon;

(3) Evidence that the person owns or leases property in Oregon; or

(4) Filing of an Oregon tax return for the most recent tax year. [1995 c.3 §3.10; 1999 c.423 §8]

127.865 §3.11. Reporting requirements. (1)(a) The Department of Human Services shall annually review a sample of records maintained pursuant to ORS 127.800 to 127.897.

(b) The department shall require any health care provider upon dispensing medication pursuant to ORS 127.800 to 127.897 to file a copy of the dispensing record with the department.

(2) The department shall make rules to facilitate the collection of information regarding compliance with ORS 127.800 to 127.897. Except as otherwise required by law, the information collected shall not be a public record and may not be made available for inspection by the public.

(3) The department shall generate and make available to the public an annual statistical report of information collected under subsection (2) of this section. [1995 c.3 §3.11; 1999 c.423 §9; 2001 c.104 §40]

127.870 §3.12. Effect on construction of wills, contracts and statutes. (1) No provision in a contract, will or other agreement, whether written or oral, to the extent the provision would affect whether a person may make or rescind a request for medication to end his or her life in a humane and dignified manner, shall be valid.

(2) No obligation owing under any currently existing contract shall be conditioned or affected by the making or rescinding of a request, by a person, for medication to end his or her life in a humane and dignified manner. [1995 c.3 §3.12]

127.875 §3.13. Insurance or annuity policies. The sale, procurement, or issuance of any life, health, or accident insurance or annuity policy or the rate charged for any policy shall not be conditioned upon or affected by the making or rescinding of a request, by a person, for medication to end his or her life in a humane and dignified manner. Neither shall a qualified patient's act of ingesting medication to end his or her life in a humane and dignified manner have an effect upon a life, health, or accident insurance or annuity policy. [1995 c.3 §3.13]

127.880 §3.14. Construction of Act. Nothing in ORS 127.800 to 127.897 shall be construed to authorize a physician or any other person to end a patient's life by lethal injection, mercy killing or active euthanasia. Actions taken in accordance with ORS 127.800 to 127.897 shall not, for any purpose, constitute suicide, assisted suicide, mercy killing or homicide, under the law. [1995 c.3 §3.14]

(Immunities and Liabilities)

(Section 4)

127.885 §4.01. Immunities; basis for prohibiting health care provider from participation; notification; permissible sanctions. Except as provided in ORS 127.890:

(1) No person shall be subject to civil or criminal liability or professional disciplinary action for participating in good faith compliance with ORS 127.800 to 127.897. This includes being present when a qualified patient

takes the prescribed medication to end his or her life in a humane and dignified manner.

(2) No professional organization or association, or health care provider, may subject a person to censure, discipline, suspension, loss of license, loss of privileges, loss of membership or other penalty for participating or refusing to participate in good faith compliance with ORS 127.800 to 127.897.

(3) No request by a patient for or provision by an attending physician of medication in good faith compliance with the provisions of ORS 127.800 to 127.897 shall constitute neglect for any purpose of law or provide the sole basis for the appointment of a guardian or conservator.

(4) No health care provider shall be under any duty, whether by contract, by statute or by any other legal requirement to participate in the provision to a qualified patient of medication to end his or her life in a humane and dignified manner. If a health care provider is unable or unwilling to carry out a patient's request under ORS 127.800 to 127.897, and the patient transfers his or her care to a new health care provider, the prior health care provider shall transfer, upon request, a copy of the patient's relevant medical records to the new health care provider.

(5) (a) Notwithstanding any other provision of law, a health care provider may prohibit another health care provider from participating in ORS 127.800 to 127.897 on the premises of the prohibiting provider if the prohibiting provider has notified the health care provider of the prohibiting provider's policy regarding participating in ORS 127.800 to 127.897. Nothing in this paragraph prevents a health care provider from providing health care services to a patient that do not constitute participation in ORS 127.800 to 127.897.

(b) Notwithstanding the provisions of subsections (1) to (4) of this section, a health care provider may subject another health care provider to the sanctions stated in this paragraph if the sanctioning health care provider has notified the sanctioned provider prior to participation in ORS 127.800 to 127.897 that it prohibits participation in ORS 127.800 to 127.897:

(A) Loss of privileges, loss of membership or other sanction provided pursuant to the medical staff bylaws, policies and procedures of the sanctioning health care provider if the sanctioned provider is a member of the sanctioning provider's medical staff and participates in ORS 127.800 to 127.897 while on the health care facility premises, as defined in ORS 442.015, of the sanctioning health care provider, but not including the private medical office of a physician or other provider;

(B) Termination of lease or other property contract or other non-monetary remedies provided by lease contract, not including loss or restriction of medical staff privileges or exclusion from a provider panel, if the sanctioned provider participates in ORS 127.800 to 127.897 while on the premises of the sanctioning health care provider or on property that is owned by or under the direct control of the sanctioning health care provider; or

(C) Termination of contract or other nonmonetary remedies provided by contract if the sanctioned provider participates in ORS 127.800 to 127.897 while acting in the course and scope of the sanctioned provider's capacity as an employee or independent contractor of the sanctioning health care provider. Nothing in this subparagraph shall be construed to prevent:

(i) A health care provider from participating in ORS 127.800 to 127.897 while acting outside the course and scope of the provider's capacity as an employee or independent contractor; or

(ii) A patient from contracting with his or her attending physician and consulting physician to act outside the course and scope of the provider's capacity as an employee or independent contractor of the sanctioning health care provider.

(d) A health care provider that imposes sanctions pursuant to paragraph (b) of this subsection must follow all due process and other procedures the sanctioning health care provider may have that are related to the imposition of sanctions on another health care provider.

(b) For purposes of this subsection:

(A) "Notify" means a separate statement in writing to the health care provider specifically informing the health care provider prior to the provider's participation in ORS 127.800 to 127.897 of the sanctioning health care provider's policy about participation in activities covered by ORS 127.800 to 127.897.

(B) "Participate in ORS 127.800 to 127.897" means to perform the duties of an attending physician pursuant to ORS 127.815, the consulting physician function pursuant to ORS 127.820 or the counseling function pursuant to ORS 127.825. "Participate in ORS 127.800 to 127.897" does not include:

(i) Making an initial determination that a patient has a terminal disease and informing the patient of the medical prognosis;

      (ii) Providing information about the Oregon Death with Dignity Act to a patient upon the request of the patient;

      (iii) Providing a patient, upon the request of the patient, with a referral to another physician; or

      (iv) A patient contracting with his or her attending physician and consulting physician to act outside of the course and scope of the provider's capacity as an employee or independent contractor of the sanctioning health care provider.

(6) Suspension or termination of staff membership or privileges under subsection (5) of this section is not reportable under ORS 441.820. Action taken pursuant to ORS 127.810, 127.815, 127.820 or 127.825 shall not be the sole basis for a report of unprofessional or dishonorable conduct under ORS 677.415 (2) or (3).

(7) No provision of ORS 127.800 to 127.897 shall be construed to allow a lower standard of care for patients in the community where the patient is treated or a similar community. [1995 c.3 §4.01; 1999 c.423 §10]

Note: As originally enacted by the people, the leadline to section 4.01 read "Immunities." The remainder of the leadline was added by editorial action.

127.890 §4.02. Liabilities. (1) A person who without authorization of the patient willfully alters or forges a request for medication or conceals or destroys a rescission of that request with the intent or effect of causing the patient's death shall be guilty of a Class A felony.

(2) A person who coerces or exerts undue influence on a patient to request medication for the purpose of ending the patient's life, or to destroy a rescission of such a request, shall be guilty of a Class A felony.

(3) Nothing in ORS 127.800 to 127.897 limits further liability for civil damages resulting from other negligent conduct or intentional misconduct by any person.

(4) The penalties in ORS 127.800 to 127.897 do not preclude criminal penalties applicable under other law for conduct which is inconsistent with the provisions of ORS 127.800 to 127.897. [1995 c.3 §4.02]

127.892 Claims by governmental entity for costs incurred. Any governmental entity that incurs costs resulting from a person terminating his or her life pursuant to the provisions of ORS 127.800 to 127.897 in a public place shall have a claim against the estate of the person to recover such costs and reasonable attorney fees related to enforcing the claim. [1999 c.423 §5a]

(Severability)

(Section 5)

127.895 §5.01. Severability. Any section of ORS 127.800 to 127.897 being held invalid as to any person or circumstance shall not affect the application of any other section of ORS 127.800 to 127.897 which can be given full effect without the invalid section or application. [1995 c.3 §5.01]

(Form of the Request) (Section 6)

127.897 §6.01. Form of the request. A request for a medication as authorized by ORS 127.800 to 127.897 shall be in substantially the following form:

REQUEST FOR MEDICATION
TO END MY LIFE IN A HUMANE
AND DIGNIFIED MANNER

I, _____, am an adult of sound mind.

I am suffering from_____, which my attending physician has determined is a terminal disease and which has been medically confirmed by a consulting physician.

I have been fully informed of my diagnosis, prognosis, the nature of medication to be prescribed and potential associated risks, the expected result, and the feasible alternatives, including comfort care, hospice care and pain control.

I request that my attending physician prescribe medication that will end my life in a humane and dignified manner.

INITIAL ONE:

_____I have informed my family of my decision and taken their opinions into consideration.

_____I have decided not to inform my family of my decision.

_____I have no family to inform of my decision.

I understand that I have the right to rescind this request at any time.

I understand the full import of this request and I expect to die when I take the medication to be prescribed. I further understand that although most deaths occur within three hours, my death may take longer and my physician has counseled me about this possibility.

I make this request voluntarily and without reservation, and I accept full moral responsibility for my actions.

Signed: _____

Dated: _____

DECLARATION OF WITNESSES

We declare that the person signing this request:

   (a) Is personally known to us or has provided proof of identity;
   (b) Signed this request in our presence;
   (c) Appears to be of sound mind and not under duress, fraud or undue influence;
   (d) Is not a patient for whom either of us is attending physician.

_____Witness 1/Date
_____Witness 2/Date

NOTE: One witness shall not be a relative (by blood, marriage or adoption) of the person signing this request, shall not be entitled to any portion of the person's estate upon death and shall not own, operate or be employed at a health care facility where the person is a patient or resident. If the patient is an inpatient at a health care facility, one of the witnesses shall be an individual designated by the facility.

_____

_____

[1995 c.3 §6.01; 1999 c.423 §11]

PENALTIES

127.990: [Formerly part of 97.990; repealed by 1993 c.767 §29]

127.995 Penalties. (1) It shall be a Class A felony for a person without authorization of the principal to willfully alter, forge, conceal or destroy an instrument, the reinstatement or revocation of an instrument or any other evidence or document reflecting the principal's desires and interests, with the intent and effect of causing a withholding or withdrawal of life-sustaining procedures or of artificially administered nutrition and hydration which hastens the death of the principal.

   (2) Except as provided in subsection (1) of this section, it shall be a Class A misdemeanor for a person without authorization of the principal to willfully alter, forge, conceal or destroy an instrument, the reinstatement or revocation of an instrument, or any other evidence or document reflecting the principal's desires and interests with the intent or effect of affecting a health care decision. [Formerly 127.585]

CONSULTING PHYSICIAN'S COMPLIANCE FORM
ORS 127.800 - ORS 127.897
Deliver this form to the attending/prescribing physician who will mail it to:
Oregon State Public Health Division, Center for Health Statistics,
P.O. Box 14050, Portland, OR 97293-0050

☞ **PLEASE PRINT**

A | **PATIENT INFORMATION**

PATIENT'S NAME (LAST, FIRST, M.I.) | DATE OF BIRTH

B | **REFERRING/PRESCRIBING PHYSICIAN**

REFERRING/PRESCRIBING PHYSICIAN'S NAME (LAST, FIRST, M.I.) | TELEPHONE NUMBER ( ) —

C | **CONSULTANT'S REPORT**

1. MEDICAL DIAGNOSIS | DATE OF EXAMINATION(S)

2. Check boxes for compliance. *(Both the attending and consulting physicians must make these determinations.)*

☐ 1. Determination that the patient has a terminal disease.
☐ 2. Determination the patient has 6 months or less to live.
☐ 3. Determination that patient is capable.**
☐ 4. Determination that patient is acting voluntarily.
5. Determination that patient has made his/her decision after being fully informed of:
☐ a. His or her medical diagnosis; and
☐ b. His or her prognosis; and
☐ c. The potential risks associated with taking the medication to be prescribed; and
☐ d. The potential result of taking the medication to be prescribed; and
☐ e. The feasible alternatives, including, but not limited to, comfort care, hospice care and pain control.
Comments:

D | **PATIENT'S MENTAL STATUS**

Check one of the following *(required)*:
☐ I have determined that the patient is not suffering from a psychiatric or psychological disorder, or depression causing impaired judgment, in conformance with ORS 127.825.
☐ I have referred the patient to the provider listed below for evaluation and counseling for a possible psychiatric or psychological disorder, or depression causing impaired judgment.

PSYCHIATRIC CONSULTANT'S NAME | TELEPHONE NUMBER ( ) — | DATE

E | **CONSULTANT'S INFORMATION**

X | PHYSICIAN'S SIGNATURE | DATE
| NAME (PLEASE PRINT)
MAILING ADDRESS
CITY, STATE AND ZIP CODE | TELEPHONE NUMBER ( ) —

** "Capable" means that in the opinion of a court or in the opinion of the patient's attending physician or consulting physician, a patient has the ability to make and communicate health care decisions to health care providers, including communication through persons familiar with the patient's manner of communicating, if those persons are available.
Note: This form is revised periodically. To assure that you are using the most current version, please refer to:
http://egov.oregon.gov/DHS/ph/pas/index.shtml

Rev. 11/06

SEND A COPY OF THIS FORM TO THE OREGON STATE PUBLIC HEALTH DIVISION
ATTENDING PHYSICIAN'S COMPLIANCE FORM
ORS 127.800 - ORS 127.897
MAIL FORM TO: Oregon State Public Health Division, Center for Health Statistics,
P.O. Box 14050, Portland, OR 97293-0050

☞ **PLEASE PRINT**

A	PATIENT INFORMATION	
PATIENT'S NAME (LAST, FIRST, M.I.)		DATE OF BIRTH:
MEDICAL DIAGNOSIS		

B	PHYSICIAN INFORMATION	
NAME (LAST, FIRST, M.I.)		TELEPHONE NUMBER ( ) —
MAILING ADDRESS		
CITY, STATE AND ZIP CODE		

C	ACTION TAKEN TO COMPLY WITH LAW	

1. FIRST ORAL REQUEST

First oral request for medication to end life.	DATE
Comments:	

Indicate compliance by checking the boxes. (Both the attending and consulting physicians must make these determinations.)

☐ 1. Determination that the patient has a terminal disease.
☐ 2. Determination the patient has six months or less to live.
☐ 3. Determination that patient is capable.**
☐ 4. Determination that patient is an Oregon resident.***
☐ 5. Determination that patient is acting voluntarily.
   6. Determination that patient has made his/her decision after being fully informed of:
☐   a) His or her medical diagnosis; and
☐   b) His or her prognosis; and
☐   c) The potential risks associated with taking the medication to be prescribed; and
☐   d) The potential result of taking the medication to be prescribed; and
☐   e) The feasible alternatives, including, but not limited to, comfort care, hospice care and pain control.

Indicate compliance by checking the boxes.   DATE:
☐ 1. Patient informed of his or her right to rescind the request at any time.
☐ 2. Patient recommended to inform next of kin.
☐ 3. Patient counseled about the importance of having another person present when the patient takes the medication(s).
☐ 4. Patient counseled about the importance of not taking the medication in a public place.

2. SECOND ORAL REQUEST *(Must be made **15 days** or more after the first oral request.)*

Indicate compliance by checking the boxes.   DATE:
☐ 1. Second oral request for medication to end life.
☐ 2. Patient informed of the right to rescind the request at any time.
Comments:

Rev. 11/06

SEND A COPY OF THIS FORM TO THE OREGON STATE PUBLIC HEALTH DIVISION
ATTENDING PHYSICIAN'S COMPLIANCE FORM (continued)

PATIENT INFORMATION

PATIENT'S NAME (LAST, FIRST, M.I.)	DATE OF BIRTH

C   **ACTION TAKEN TO COMPLY WITH THE LAW – continued**

3. PATIENT'S WRITTEN REQUEST

☐ Written request for medication to end life received. Please attach request. *(No less than 48 hours shall elapse between the written request and writing the prescription.)*	DATE

Comments:

D   **MEDICAL CONSULTATION (Attach consultant's form.)**

Medical consultation and second opinion requested from:

MEDICAL CONSULTANT'S NAME	TELEPHONE NUMBER ( ) —	DATE

E   **PSYCHIATRIC/PSYCHOLOGICAL EVALUATION**

Check one of the following (required):

☐ I have determined that the patient is not suffering from a psychiatric or psychological disorder, or depression, causing impaired judgment, in accordance with ORS 127.825.

☐ I have referred the patient to the provider listed below for evaluation and counseling for a possible psychiatric or psychological disorder, or depression causing impaired judgment, **and attached the consultant's form.**

PSYCHIATRIC CONSULTANT'S NAME	TELEPHONE NUMBER ( ) —	DATE

F   **MEDICATION PRESCRIBED AND INFORMATION PROVIDED TO PATIENT**
*(To be prescribed no sooner than **48 hours** after patient's written request has been signed.)*

Lethal medication prescribed *and dose*	DATE PRESCRIBED

Please check one of the following:

☐ Dispensed medication directly. Date ____/____/____

☐ Contacted pharmacist and delivered prescription personally or by mail to the pharmacist.

Pharmacy Name   City   Phone # ( ) -

Immediately prior to writing the prescription, the patient was fully informed of: *(check boxes)*

☐ (a) his or her medical diagnosis;

☐ (b) his or her prognosis;

☐ (c) the potential risks associated with taking the medication to be prescribed;

☐ (d) the probable result of taking the medication to be prescribed;

☐ (e) the feasible alternatives, including, but not limited to, comfort care, hospice care and pain control.

To the best of my knowledge, all of the requirements under the Death with Dignity Act have been met.

✗ PHYSICIAN'S SIGNATURE	DATE

* If comments in any section exceed the space provided, please use an attached page. Supplemental comments should be identified using the appropriate alpha-numeric notation (e.g., C3).

** "Capable" means that in the opinion of a court, or in the opinion of the patient's attending physician or consulting physician, a patient has the ability to make and communicate health care decisions to health care providers, including communication through persons familiar with the patient's manner of communicating, if those persons are available.

*** Factors demonstrating residency include, but are not limited to: 1) Possession of an Oregon driver's license; 2) Registration to vote in Oregon; 3) Evidence that a person leases/owns property in Oregon; or 4) Filing of an Oregon tax return for the most recent tax year. Only the attending physician is required to affirm Oregon residency.

*Note: Besides this form, **it is the attending physician's responsibility** to send the following documents to the Public Health Division: 1) Patient's written request; 2) Consulting physician's report; and 3) Psychiatric evaluation referral report (if performed).*

This form is revised periodically. To assure that you are using the most current version, please refer to:
http://egov.oregon.gov/DHS/ph/pas/index.shtml

Rev. 11/06

NOTES

Chapter 1

1. Margaret Pabst Battin, *Ending Life: Ethics and the Way We Die* (New York: Oxford University Press, 2005), p. 94. See also Steven M. Miles, *The Hippocratic Oath and the Ethics of Medicine* (New York: Oxford University Press, 2004).
2. Seneca, Ep. Lxx, cited by W.H.E. Lecky, *History of European Morals from Augustus to Charlemagne* (New York: George Braziller, 1955), vol. 1, p. 218.
3. Letter 70 to Lucilius, cited by Battin, *Ending Life*, p. 4.
4. For a fuller discussion, see David Novak, *Suicide and Morality: The Theories of Plato, Aquinas and Kant and Their Relevance to Suicidology* (New York: Scholars Studies Press, 1975), and Robert W. Wennberg, *Terminal Choices: Euthanasia, Suicide, and the Right to Die* (Grand Rapids, MI: William B. Eerdmans, 1989).
5. Jim Persels, "Forcing the Issue of Physician-assisted Suicide," *Journal of Legal Medicine* 14 (1993):101. For a good history of the right-to-die movement, see Ian Dowbiggin, *A Merciful End: The Euthanasia Movement in Modern America* (New York: Oxford University Press, 2003.
6. For a good discussion of the fallacies involved in the slippery-slope argument, see Margaret Pabst Battin, *The Least Worst Death: Essays in Bioethics on the End of Life* (New York: Oxford University Press, 1994), pp. 20–24.
7. Park Ridge Center for the Study of Health, Faith and Ethics, *Active Euthanasia, Religion, and the Public Debate* (Chicago: Park Ridge Center, 1991), p. 32.
8. Melvin I. Urofsky, *Lethal Judgments: Assisted Suicide and American Law* (Lawrence: University Press of Kansas, 2000), p. 34.
9. *Cruzan v. Director, Missouri Department of Health*, 497 U.S. 261 (1990). See also *In the Matter of Karen Quinlan*, 70 N.J. 10, 355 A.2nd 647 (1976).
10. 42 U.S.C. 1395 cc (a).

11. Barry Rosenfeld, *Assisted Suicide and the Right to Die: The Interface of Social Science, Public Policy and Medical Ethics* (Washington, DC: American Psychological Association, 2004), pp. 51–54.

12. Robert S. Olick, *Taking Advance Directives Seriously: Prospective Autonomy and Decisions Near the End of Life* (Washington, DC: Georgetown University Press, 2001), pp. 27, 168–69.

13. Timothy Quill and Diane E. Meier, "The Big Chill: Inserting the DEA into End-of-Life Care," *New England Journal of Medicine* 354 (2006): 1–2.

14. Charles H. Baron, "Hastening Death: The Seven Deadly Sins of the Status Quo," in *Physician-assisted Dying: The Case for Palliative Care and Patient Choice*, edited by Timothy E. Quill and Margaret P. Battin (Baltimore, MD: Johns Hopkins University Press, 2004), p. 317.

15. *Washington v. Glucksberg*, 521 U.S. 702 (1997) and *Vacco v. Quill*, 521 U.S. 193 (1997).

16. *Robert Baxter et al. v. State of Montana*, 2008 Mont. Dist. LEXIS 482.

17. Kirk Johnson, "Ruling by Montana Supreme Court Bolsters Physician-Assisted Suicide," *New York Times*, January 1, 2010.

18. Carol Poenisch, "Meriam Frederick's Story," *New England Journal of Medicine* 339 (1998): 996–98.

19. Cf. Quill and Battin, eds., *Physician-assisted Dying*, Introduction, p. 5. See also Silvia Sara Canetto and Janet D. Hollenshead, "Gender and Physician-assisted Suicide: An Analysis of the Kevorkian Cases, 1990–1997," *Omega: The Journal of Death and Dying* 40 (1999–2000): 165–208, who show that almost half of 75 analyzed Kevorkian cases involved ALS or multiple sclerosis.

20. "It's Over, Debbie," *Journal of the American Medical Association* 259 (1988): 272.

21. News release of November 5, 2008, www.finalexitnetwork.org. Accessed January 15, 2010.

22. Jane E. Brody, "Terminal Options for the Irreversibly Ill," *New York Times*, March 18, 2008.

23. Urofsky, *Lethal Judgments*, p. 73.

24. Final Exit Network news release, February 26, 2009.

25. Greg Bluestein, "Assisted Suicide Presents Legal Quandary," *Washington Post*, March 2, 2009.

26. Margaret P. Battin, "New Life in the Assisted Death Debate in the United States: Scheduled Drugs and NuTech," in *Regulating Physician-Negotiated Death*, edited by Albert Klijn et al. (s'Gravenhage: Elsevier, 2001), p. 56; Russell D. Ogden, "Non-Physician Assisted Suicide: The Technological Imperative of the Deathing Counterculture," *Death Studies* 25 (2001):398.

27. Lance K. Stell, "Physician-assisted Suicide: To Decriminalize or to Legalize, That is the Question," in *Physician-assisted Suicide: Expanding the Debate*, edited by Margaret P. Battin et al. (New York: Routledge, 1998), p. 225.

28. Battin, *Ending Life*, pp. 23–24.

29. See the contrasting views of Timothy E. Quill, "Palliative Treatments of Last Resort: Choosing the Least Harmful Alternative," *Annals of Internal Medicine* 132 (2000): 491–92, and Clay W. Jackson, "Palliative Sedation vs. Terminal Sedation: What's in a Name," *American Journal of Hospice and Palliative Care* 19 (2002): 81–82.

30. The issues of the distinction between killing and letting die as well as the doctrine of the double effect are well-discussed in Battin, *The Least Worst Death: Introduction*.

31. Ezekiel J. Emanuel, "Euthanasia and Physician-assisted Suicide: A Review of the Empirical Data from the United States," *Archives of Internal Medicine* 162 (2002): 145–150.

32. Ezekiel J. Emanuel et al., "Euthanasia and Physician-assisted Suicide: Attitudes and Experiences of Oncology Patients, Oncologists and the Public," *The Lancet* 347 (1996): 1808.

33. Anthony Back et al., "Physician-assisted Suicide and Euthanasia in Washington State: Patient Requests and Physician Responses," *Journal of the American Medical Association* 275 (1996): 920–22.

34. Diane E. Meier et al., "A National Survey of Physician-assisted Suicide and Euthanasia in the United States," *New England Journal of Medicine* 338 (1998): 1195.

35. Marianne La Porte Matzo and Ezekiel J. Emanuel, "Oncology Nurses' Practices of Assisted Suicide and Patient-Requested Euthanasia," *Oncology Nursing Forum* 24 (1997): 1729.

36. Timothy E. Quill et al., "The Debate over Physician-assisted Suicide: Empirical Data and Convergent Views," *Annals of Internal Medicine* 128 (1998): 554.

37. Timothy E. Quill. *A Midwife Through the Dying Process: Stories of Healing and Hard Choices at the End of Life* (Baltimore, MD: Johns Hopkins University Press, 1996), p. 214.

38. Roger S. Magnusson, *Angels of Death: Exploring the Euthanasia Underground* (New Haven, CT: Yale University Press, 2002), p. 201.

39. Kathy Faber-Langendoen and Jason H.T. Karlawish, "Ought Assisted Suicide Be Only Physician-assisted?" in *Assisted Suicide: Finding Common Ground*, edited by Lois Snyder and Arthur L. Kaplan (Bloomington, IN: Indiana University Press, 2002), p. 49.

40. Magnusson, *Angels of Death*, pp. 246, 198.

41. David A. Asch, "The Role of Critical Care Nurses in Euthanasia and Assisted Suicide," *New England Journal of Medicine* 334 (1996): 1376.

42. Back et al., "Physician-assisted Suicide and Euthanasia in Washington State," p. 925.

43. Meier et al., "A National Survey of Physician-assisted Suicide and Euthanasia," p. 1200.

44. Nico N. Peruzzi et al., "Physician-assisted Suicide: The Role of Mental Health Professionals," *Ethics and Behavior* 6 (1996): 354.

45. Rosenfeld, *Assisted Suicide and the Right to Die*, p. 91.

46. Ibid., p. 123; Mark D. Sullivan, "Should Psychiatrists Serve as Gatekeepers for Physician-assisted Suicide?" *Hastings Center Reports*, vol. 28, no. 4 (July-August 1998): 27–28.

47. Susan D. Block and J. Andrew Billings, "Patient Requests for Euthanasia and Assisted Suicide in Terminal Illness: The Role of the Psychiatrist," *Psychosomatics* 36 (1995): 448.

48. See, e.g., Ezekiel J. Emanuel et al., "Attitudes and Desires Related to Euthanasia and Physician-assisted Suicide Among Terminally Ill Patients and Their Caregivers," *Journal of the American Medical Association* 284 (2000): 2467.

49. Karen Blank et al., "Instability of Attitudes about Euthanasia and Physician-assisted Suicide in Depressed Older Hospitalized Patients," *General Hospital Psychiatry* 23 (2001): 330–31.

50. Neil M. Gorsuch, *The Future of Assisted Suicide and Euthanasia* (Princeton, NJ: Princeton University Press, 2006), p. 137.

51. Margaret Otlowski, 'The Effectiveness of Legal Control of Euthanasia: Lessons from Comparative Law," in *Regulating Physician-Negotiated Death*, edited by Klijn et al., p. 154.

52. Barry Rosenfeld, "Assisted Suicide, Depression, and the Right to Die," *Psychology, Public Policy, and Law* 6 (2000): 479.

53. "Declaration on Euthanasia," May 5, 1980, online statement by Adoremus, the Society for the Renewal of the Sacred Liturgy. Available at www.adoremus.org. Accessed January 15, 2010.

54. Gorsuch, *The Future of Assisted Suicide and Euthanasia*, p. 157.

55. For a good discussion of the moral issues, see Linda L. Emanuel, "A Question of Balance," in *Regulating How We Die: The Ethical, Medical, and Legal Issues Surrounding Physician-assisted Suicide*, edited by Linda L. Emanuel (Cambridge, MA: Harvard University Press, 1998), pp. 234–48.

56. Ibid., pp. 138–39.

57. Task Force on Physician-assisted Suicide, "Physician-assisted Suicide: Towards a Comprehensive Understanding," *Academic Medicine* 70 (1995): 588.

58. Johannes M. van Delden. Slippery Slopes in Flat Countries: A Response," *Journal of Medical Ethics* 25 (1999): 24.

Chapter 2

1. Jacob J.F. Visser and Herman H. van der Kloot Meijburg, "The Long Road to Legalizing Physician-assisted Death in the Netherlands," *Illness, Crisis and Loss* 11 (2003): 114.
2. J.H. van den Berg, *Medische macht en medische ethiek* (Nijkerk, 1969); an English translation, *Medical Power and Medical Ethics*, was published by W.W. Norton in 1978.
3. John Griffiths et al., *Euthanasia and Law in the Netherlands* (Amsterdam: Amsterdam University Press, 1998), pp. 54–56.
4. David C. Thomasma et al., *Asking to Die: Inside the Dutch Debate About Euthanasia* (Dortrecht: Kluwer Academic Publishers, 1998), pp. 7–8.
5. Griffiths, *Euthanasia and Law*, pp. 58–60.
6. Ibid., pp. 62–63, 99. The decision is reprinted on pp. 322–28.
7. "Guidelines for Euthanasia," *Issues in Law and Medicine* 3 (1988): 429–37.
8. Griffiths et al., *Euthanasia and Law*, pp. 69–72. This book reproduces the full report in appendix I-C-1 (pp. 314–16).
9. Ibid., pp. 66–67.
10. Ibid., pp. 74–75; Johan Legemaate, "Twenty-five Years of Dutch Experience and Policy on Euthanasia and Assisted Suicide: An Overview," in Thomasma et al., *Asking to Die*, pp. 24–25.
11. Griffiths et al., *Euthanasia and Law*, p. 77.
12. Legemaate, "Twenty-five Years of Dutch Experience," p. 84.
13. Ibid., pp. 79–80. The text of the law and of the "points requiring attention" is reproduced in Griffiths et al., *Euthanasia and Law*, appendix I-B (pp. 308–13).
14. Jacqueline M. Cuperus-Bosma, "Physician-assisted Death: Policy-making by the Assembly of Procurators-General in the Netherlands," *European Journal of Health Law* 4 (1997): 226.
15. Ibid., Jacqueline M. Cuperus-Bosma, "Assessment of Physician-assisted Death by Members of the Public Prosecution in the Netherlands," *Journal of Medical Ethics* 25 (1999): 13.
16. Legemaate, "Twenty-five Years of Dutch Experience," p. 30.
17. Gerrit van der Wal et al., "Euthanasia and Assisted Suicide. II. Do Dutch Family Doctors Act Prudently?" *Family Practice* 9 (1992): 138.
18. Marijke Catharina Jansen-van der Weide et al., "Implementation of the Project 'Support and Consultation in the Netherlands' (SCEN)," *Health Policy* 69 (2004): 366–67.

19. Van der Wal et al., "Euthanasia and Assisted Suicide. II," p. 138.
20. Ibid., pp. 368–71. Marijke Catharina Jansen-van der Weide et al., "Quality of Consultation and the Project 'Support and Consultation on Euthanasia in the Netherlands' (SCEN)," *Health Policy* 80 (2007): 105–106.
21. For a detailed account of developments leading up to the introduction of this bill and its key provisions, see "Bill on Euthanasia and Assisting Suicide in the Netherlands," *European Journal of Health Law* 5 (1998): 299–324.
22. *Staatsblad* 2001: 1–8. I have used the official English translation reproduced in Paul Schotsmans and Tom Meulenberg, eds., *Euthanasia and Palliative Care in the Low Countries* (Leuven, BE: Peeters, 2005). The full text of the law can be found in Appendix 1 of the present work (pp. 161–71).
23. The forms to be used by physicians are reprinted in Antonia Grundmann, *Das niederländische Gesetz über die Prüfung von Lebensbeendigung auf Verlangen und Beihilfe zur Selbsttötung* (Aachen: Shaker, 2004), pp. 225–30.
24. Paul van der Maas et al., *Euthanasia and Other Medical Decisions Concerning the End of Life: A Investigation* (Amsterdam: Elsevier, 1992); Paul J. van der Maas et al., "Euthanasia and Other Medical Decisions Converning the End of Life," *Health Policy* 22 (1992): Special issue, pp. 1–262. A summary of the report, under the same title, appeared in *The Lancet* (1991): 669–74.
25. Paul J. van der Maas et al., "Euthanasia, Physician-assisted suicide, and Other Medical Practices Involving the End of Life in the Netherlands: 1990–1995," *New England Journal of Medicine* 335 (1996): 1699–1705; Gerrit van der Wal and P.J. van der Maas, "Empirical Research on Euthanasia and Other Medical End-of-Life Decisions and the Euthanasia Notification Procedure," in Thomasma et al., *Asking to Die*, pp. 150–51; Gerritt van der Wal et al., *Medische besluitvorming aan het einde van het leven: De paraktijk en de toet-singsprocedure euthanasia* [Medical Decision-making at the End of Life: The Practice and Euthanasia Procedure] (Utrecht: Uitgeverij de Tijdstrom, 2003). I have used the summary of the 2001–2002 report in Grundmann, *Das niederländische Gesetz über die Prüfung von Lebensbeendigung auf Verlangen und Beihilfe zur Selbsttötung*, pp. 203–214; Agnes van der Heide et al., "End-of-Life Practices in the Netherlands Under the Euthanasia Act," *New England Journal of Medicine* 356 (2007): 1957–1965.
26. Netherlands Ministry of Health, Welfare and Sport, *Evaluation-Summary: Termination of the Life on Request and Assisted Suicide (Review Procedures) Act* by Bregje D. Onwuteaka-Philipsen et al. (May 22, 2007), Available at http://www.minvws.nl/themes/euthanasia; accessed January 17, 2010.
27. Paul J. van der Maas, "Euthanasia and Other Medical Decisions Concerning the End of Life," *The Lancet* 338 (1991): 669–70.
28. Netherlands Ministry of Health, Welfare and Sport, *Evaluation-Summary* by Onwuteaka-Philipsen et al. (May 22, 2007), p. 7; Netherlands, Regional

Euthanasia Review Committees, 2006 annual report (May 2007), p. 11. Available at http://toetsingscommissieseuthanasie.nl/en; accessed January 17, 2010 (English version).

29. Ilinka Haverkate et al., "Refused and Granted Requests for Euthanasia and Assisted Suicide in the Netherlands: Interview Study with Structured Questionnaire," *British Medical Journal* 321 (2000): 866.

30. Marijke C. Jansen-van der Weide et al., "Granted, Undecided, Withdrawn, and Refused Requests for Euthanasia and Physician-assisted Suicide," p. 1702.

31. Haverkate et al., "Refused and Granted Requests for Euthanasia and Assisted Suicide," p. 866.

32. Thomasma et al., *Asking to Die*, p. 12.

33. Van der Maas et al., "Euthanasia, Physician-assisted Suicide, and Other Medical Practices Involving the End of Life in the Netherlands," p. 1704.

34. Van der Heide et al., "End-of-Life Practices in the Netherlands Under the Euthanasia Act," p. 1963.

35. Van der Maas et al., "Euthanasia and Other Medical Decisions Concerning the End of Life," p. 672.

36. Jansen-van der Weide et al., "Granted, Undecided, Withdrawn, and Refused Requests for Euthanasia and Physician-assisted Suicide," p. 1700.

37. Netherlands, Regional Euthanasia Review Committees, 2006 annual report, p. 11.

38. Van der Maas et al., "Euthanasia and Other Medical Decisions Concerning the End of Life," p. 673.

39. Agnes Rietjens et al., "Preferences of the Dutch General Public for a Good Death and Associations with Attitudes Towards End-of-Life Decisions," *Palliative Medicine* 20 (2006): 689.

40. Grundmann, *Das niederländische Gesetz über die Prüfung von Lebensbeendigung auf Verlangen*, p. 213.

41. P. Kohnen and G. Schumacher, eds., *Euthanasia and Human Dignity: A Collection of Contributions by the Dutch Catholic Bishops' Conference to the Legislative Procedure 1983–2001* (Utrecht/Leuven: Peeters, 2002), p. 161.

42. Hans Küng et al., *Dying with Dignity: A Plea for Personal Responsibility* (New York: Continuum, 1995), p. 115.

43. Jenny T. van der Steen et al., "End-of-Life Decision Making in Nursing Home Residents with Dementia and Pneumonia: Dutch Physicians' Intentions regarding Hastening of Death," *Alzheimer Disease and Associated Disorders* 19 (2005): 150–152.

44. Haverkate and G. van der Wal, "Dutch Nursing Home Policies and Guidelines on Physician-assisted death and Decisions to Forego Treatment," *Public Health* 112 (1998): 420–21.

45. Griffiths et al., *Euthanasia and Law*, pp. 203, 206, 249–50. The authors note that the honoring of requests for euthanasia and PAS varied considerably, from 47% in 1986 to 35% in 1989. According to the Remmelink report, less than one-third of such requests are granted (van der Maas, "Euthanasia and Other Medical Decisions Concerning the End of Life," p. 672).

46. H.S. Lau et al., "A Nationwide Study on the Practice of Euthanasia and Physician-assisted Suicide in Community Hospital Pharmacies in the Netherlands," *Pharmacy World and Science* 22 (2000): 5.

47. Ibid., pp. 3–9; Bregje D. Onwuteaka-Philipsen et al., "Euthanatics: Implementation of a Protocol to Standardize Euthanatics Among Pharmacists and GPs," *Patient Education and Counseling* 31 (1997): 132. See also the 2007 advisory report of the Royal Dutch Pharmaceutical Society, "Standard Euthanatics: Application and Preparation."

48. Griffiths et al., *Euthanasia and Law*, p. 112; Onwuteaka-Philipsen et al., "Euthanatics," pp. 131–37; Johanna H. Groenewoud et al., "Clinical Problems with the Performance of Euthanasia and Physician-assisted Suicide in the Netherlands," *New England Journal of Medicine* 342 (2000): 551–56.

49. Griffiths et al., *Euthanasia and Law*, p. 237; Bregje D. Onwuteaka-Philipsen et al., "Dutch Experience of Monitoring Euthanasia," *British Medical Journal* 331 (2005): 692.

50. Van der Wal and Van der Maas, "Empirical Research on Euthanasia and Other Medical End-of-Life Decisions," in Thomasma et al., *Asking to Die*, p. 161.

51. Albert Klijn, "Will Doctors' Behaviour Be More Accountable Under the New Dutch Regime? Reporting and Consultations as Forms of Legal Control," in *Regulating Physician-Negotiated Death*, edited by Albert Klijn et al. (s'Gravenhage: Elsevier, 2001), p. 174.

52. Griffiths et al., *Euthanasia and Law*, p. 283.

53. Van der Heide et al., "End-of-Life Practices in the Netherlands Under the Euthanasia Act," p. 1961.

54. Timothy E. Quill, *"A Midwife Through the Dying Process" Stories of Healing and Hard Choices at the End of Life* (Baltimore. MD: Johns Hopkins University Press, 1996), p. 211.

55. Griffiths et al., *Euthanasia and Law*, p. 255.

56. Evaluation-Summary by Onwuteaka-Philipsen et al., pp. 15, 17.

57. Thomasma et al., *Asking to Die*, pp. 290–91, 496.

58. Gerrit van der Wal et al., "Evaluation of the Notification Procedures for Physician-assisted Death in the Netherlands," *New England Medical Journal* 335 (1996): 1708.

59. Thomasma et al., *Asking to Die*, p. 317.

60. Klijn, "Will Doctors' Behaviour Be More Accountable Under the New Dutch Regime?," p. 162.

61. Thomasma et al., *Asking to Die*, p.13. See also Griffiths et al., *Euthanasia and Law*, pp. 205, 226–27.

62. Van der Heide et al., "End-of-Life Practices in the Netherlands Under the Euthanasia Act," pp. 1960, 1963.

63. Judith A.C. Rietjens et al., "Using Drugs to End Life Without an Explicit Request of the Patient," *Death Studies* 31 (2007): 212.

64. Pijnenborg et al., "Life-terminating Acts Without the Explicit Request of Patient," p. 1198.

65. Griffiths et al., *Euthanasia and Law*, pp. 96–97.

66. Grundmann, *Das niederländische Gesetz über die Prüfung von Lebensbeendigung*, p. 210. According to Loes Pijnenborg et al., "Life-terminating Acts without the Explicit Request of Patient," *The Lancet* 341 (1993): 1198, 36% were considered competent. The difference between these two figures may involve the distinction between the categories "competent" and "fully competent."

67. Johanna H. Groenewoud et al., "A Nationwide Study of Decisions to Forego Life-prolonging Treatment in Dutch Medical Practice," *Archives of Internal Medicine* 160 (2000): 362.

68. Rietjens et al., "Using Drugs to End Life Without an Explicit Request of the Patient," p. 214.

69. Griffiths et al., *Euthanasia and Law*, p. 239.

70. Johannes J. M. van Delden, "Slippery Slopes in Flat Countries – A Response," *Journal of Medical Ethics* 25 (1999): 24.

71. The best-known proponent of this thesis is John Keown. See his *Euthanasia, Ethics and Public Policy: An Argument Against Legalisation* (Cambridge: Cambridge University Press, 2002).

72. Pijnenborg et al., "Life-terminating Acts Without the Explicit Request of Patient," p. 1199.

73. Gerrit van der Wal, "Unrequested Termination of Life: Is It Permissible?" *Bioethics* 7 (1993): 339.

74. Summary of the 1992 report by Louis A.A. Kollée, "Current Concepts and Future Research on End-of-Life Decision Making in Neonatology in the Netherlands," in *Clinical and Epidemiological Aspects of End-of-Life Decision-Making*, edited by Agnes van der Heide et al. (Amsterdam: Royal Dutch Academy of Arts and Sciences, 2001), pp. 186–87.

75. Ibid., p. 187.

76. Griffiths et al., *Euthanasia and Law*, p. 83.

77. Ibid., pp. 83–84; Keown, *Euthanasia, Ethics and Public Policy*, p. 120.

78. Kollée, "Current Concepts and Future Research on End-of-Life Decision Making in Neonatology," p. 194.

79. Eduard Verhagen and Pieter J.J. Sauer, "The Groningen Protocol – Euthanasia in Severely Ill Newborns," *New England Medical Journal* 352 (2005): 959–62.

80. Ibid., p. 961.

81. Agnes van der Heide et al., "Medical End-of-Life Decisions Made for Neonates and Infants in the Netherlands," *The Lancet* 350 (1997): 253.

82. Ministry of Health, Welfare and Sport, press release, November 29, 2005.

83. Henk Jochemsen, "Life-prolonging and Life-terminating Treatment of Severely Handicapped Newborn Babies," *Issues in Law and Medicine* 8 (1992): 170. There is no reason to assume that Jochemsen has changed his strongly worded negative position.

84. Heide et al., "Medical End-of-Life Decisions Made for Neonates and Infants," p. 254.

85. Grundmann, *Das niederländische Gesetz über die Prüfung von Lebensbeendigung*, p. 206.

86. Avaliable at http://toetsingscommissieseuthanasie.nl/en (English version), p. 4; accessed January 17, 2010.

87. Quoted in Griffiths et al., *Euthanasia and Law*, pp. 144, 146.

88. Quoted in ibid., p. 145.

89. Ibid., p. 148.

90. Robert A. Schoevers et al., "Physician-assisted Suicide in Psychiatry: Developments in the Netherlands," *Psychiatric Services* 49 (1998): 1476; Griffiths et al., *Euthanasia and Law*, p. 81.

91. Quoted in ibid., p. 82. See also Sjef Gevers and Johan Legemaate, "Physician-assisted Suicide in Psychiatry: An Analysis of Case Law and Professional Opinions," in Thomasma et al., *Asking to Die*, p. 78.

92. Ibid.; Griffiths et al., *Euthanasia and Law*, p. 151.

93. Richard Huxtable and Maaike Möller, "'Setting a Principled Boundary'? Euthanasia as a Response to 'Life Fatigue,'" *Bioethics* 21 (2007): 118.

94. Ibid., pp. 118–19; Grundmann, *Das niederländische Gesetz über die Prüfung von Lebensbeendigung*, p. 200.

95. Gerrit K. Kimsma and Evert van Leeuwen, "Shifts in the Direction of Dutch Bioethics: Forward or Backward?" *Cambridge Quarterly of Health care Ethics* 14 (2005): 295–96.

96. Huxtable and Möller, "'Setting a Principled Boundary'?" pp. 124–25.

97. This study is discussed in Sjaak van der Geest and Anne-Marie Niekamp, "Ageism and Euthanasia in the Netherlands: Questions and Conjectures," *Mortality* 8 (2003): 297.

98. Griffiths et al., *Euthanasia and Law*, p. 82; Grundmann, *Das niederländische Gesetz über die Prüfung von Lebensbeendigung*, p. 211–12.

99. Ibid., p. 191.

100. Johanna H. Groenewoud et al., "Physician-assisted Death in Psychiatric Practice in the Netherlands," *New England Journal of Medicine* 336 (1997): 1796.

101. Schoevers et al., "Physician-assisted Suicide in Psychiatry," p. 1477.

102. Jansen-van der Weide et al., "Granted, Undecided, Withdrawn, and Refused Requests for Euthanasia and Physician-assisted Suicide," p. 1703.

103. Marije L. van der Lee et al., "Euthanasia and Depression: A Prospective Cohort Study Among Terminally Ill Cancer Patients," *Journal of Clinical Oncology* 23 (2005): 6610.

104. Johanna H. Groenewood et al., "Psychiatric Consulation with Regard to Requests for Euthanasia or Physician-assisted Suicide," *General Hospital Psychiatry* 26 (2004): 323.

105. Lee et al., "Euthanasia and Depression: A Prospective Cohort Study," p. 6611; Marjolein Bannink, "Psychiatric Consultation and Quality of Life Decision Making in Euthanasia," *The Lancet* 356 (2000): 2068.

106. Ministry of Foreign Affairs, "Questions and Answers: Euthanasia 2001." Available at www.faq-euth-2001-en[1].pdf; accessed January 17, 2010.

107. A.J.F.M. Kerkhof, "How to Deal with Requests for Assisted Suicide: Some Experiences and Practical Guidelines from the Netherlands," *Psychology, Public Policy, and Law* 6 (2000): 457, 464, 452–53.

108. Maurice Adams and Herman Nys, "Euthanasia in the Low Countries: Comparative Reflections on the Belgian and Dutch Euthanasia Act," in Schotsmans and Meulenberg, eds., *Euthanasia and Palliative Care in the Low Countries*, p. 25

109. Johannes Delden, "The Unfeasability of Requests for Euthanasia in Advance Directives," *Journal of Medical Ethics* 30 (2004): 448.

110. Doyle D. Hanks, ed., *Oxcford Textbook of Palliative Medicine* (Oxford: OUP, 1996), pp. 3–8, quoted in Rien J.P. Janssens et al., "Hospice and Euthanasia in the Netherlands: An Ethical Point of View," *Journal of Medical Ethics* 25 (1999): 408.

111. Ibid., p. 412.

112. See, e.g., the case of a patient with inoperable carcinoma of the stomach with extensive metastases, whose dispnoea and other afflictions did not yield to palliative sedation, described in the 2006 report of the Regional Review Committees. Available at http://toetsingscommissieseuthanasie.nl/en (English version, pp. 23–24); accessed January 17, 2010.

113. Rietjens et al., "Preferences of the Dutch General Public for a Good Death," pp. 689–90; Delden, "Slippery Slopes in Flat Countries," p. 23.

114. Bert Gordijn and Rien Janssens, "Euthanasia and Palliative Care in the Netherlands: An Analysis of the Latest Developments," *Health Care Analysis*

12 (2004): 199. See also the report of Anneke L. Francke, "Palliative Care for Terminally Ill Patients in the Netherlands" (Ministry of Health, Welfare and Sport publication no. 16, The Hague, 2003.)

115. Bert Broeckart and Rien Janssens, "Palliative Care and Euthanasia: Belgian and Dutch Perspectives," in *Euthanasia and Palliative Care in the Low Countries*, edited by Schotsmans and Meulenbergs, pp. 36–38.

116. Janssens et al., "Hospice and Euthanasia in the Netherlands," p. 410.

117. The existence of this sentiment is reported by Gordijn and Janssens, "Euthanasia and Palliative Care in the Netherlands," p. 202.

118. Henk Ten Have, "End-of-Life Decision Making in the Netherlands," in *End-of-Life Decision Making: A Cross-National Study*, edited by Robert H. Blank and Janna C. Merrick (Cambridge, MA: MIT Press, 2005), p. 165. Similar sentiments were expressed by several interviewees of Raphael Cohen-Almagor and reported in his article "Dutch Perspectives on Palliative Care in the Netherlands," *Issues in Law and Medicine* 18 (2002): 117–18. See also Zbigniew Zylicz, "Palliative Care and Euthanasia in the Netherlands: Observations of a Dutch Physician," in *The Case Against Assisted Suicide: For the Right to End-of-Life Care*, edited by Kathleen Foley and Herbert Hendin (Baltimore, MD: Johns Hopkins University Press, 2002), pp. 199–200.

119. Jean-Jacques Georges et al., "Physicians' Opinion on Palliative Care and Euthanasia in the Netherlands," *Journal of Palliative Care* 9 (2006): 1138.

120. Gordijn and Janssens, "Euthanasia and Palliative Care in the Netherlands," p. 199.

121. Annemieke Kuin et al., "Palliative Care Consultation in the Netherlands: A Nationwide Evaluation Study," *Journal of Pain and Symptom Management* 27 (2004): 54, 56. The budget figures are given by Gordijn and Janssens, "Euthanasia and Palliative Care in the Netherlands," p. 199.

122. Ibid., pp. 199–200; Francke, "Palliative Care for Terminally Ill Patients in the Netherlands," pp. 16–17. For the activities of Agora, see the web site www.palliatief.nl and the 2005 report of the EAPC Task Force on the Development of Palliative Care in Europe, http://www.eapcnet.org/Policy/CountriesReport.htm.

123. Francke, "Palliative Care for Terminally Ill Patients in the Netherlands," pp. 5–9.

124. Rurik Löfmark et al., "Palliative Training: A Survey of Physicians in Australia and Europe," *Journal of Palliative Care* 22 (2006): 106–107.

125. Georges et al., "Physicians' Opinion on Palliative Care and Euthanasia in the Netherlands," p. 1138.

126. Gordijn and Janssens, "Euthanasia and Palliative Care in the Netherlands," p. 200; Broeckart and Rien Janssens, "Palliative Care and Euthanasia: Belgian

and Dutch Perspectives," in *Euthanasia and Palliative Care in the Low Countries*, edited by Schotsmans and Meulenbergs, p. 42

127. Grundmann, *Das niederländische Gesetz über die Prüfung von Lebensbeendigung*, p. 211.

128. Judith Rietjens et al., "Continuous Deep Sedation for Patients Nearing Death in the Netherlands: Descriptive Study," *British Medical Journal* 336 (2008): 810–13. (I have used the online edition, March 14, 2008, pp. 1–7.)

129. Heide et al., "End-of-Life Practices in the Netherlands Under the Euthanasia Act," pp. 1962–63.

130. Tony Sheldon, "'Terminal Sedation' Different from Euthanasia, Dutch Ministers Agree," *British Medical Journal* 327 (2003): 465.

131. Gordijn and Janssens, "Euthanasia and Palliative Care in the Netherlands," p. 205, 207; Rietjens et al., "Continuous Deep Sedation for Patients Nearing Death in the Netherlands," p. 6.

132. Ibid., p. 203; Henk ten Have and Rien Janssens, *Palliative Care in Europe: Concepts and Policies* (Amsterdam: IOS Press, 2001), pp. 21–23.

133. See, e.g., the January 2007 issue of their magazine on the organization's web site http://www.nvve.nl/nvve2/pagina.asp?pagkey=72083.

134. Robert Poole, *Negotiating a Good Death: Euthanasia in the Netherlands* (New York: Haworth Press, 2000), pp. 232–33.

135. Georges et al., "Physicians' Opinion on Palliative Care and Euthanasia in the Netherlands," p. 1139.

136. Broeckart and Janssens, "Palliative Care and Euthanasia," p. 41.

137. The acceptance of this conclusion by Margaret Otlowski in her book *Voluntary Euthanasia and the Common Law* (Oxford: Clarendon Press, 1997), p. 453, was probably premature, but subsequent developments appear to have vindicated her judgment.

138. Delden, "Slippery Slopes in Flat Countries," p. 24.

139. Herbert Hendin, *Seduced by Death: Doctors, Patients, and the Dutch Cure* (New York: W.W. Norton, 1997), pp. 23, 14.

140. Herbert Hendin, "The Dutch Experience," *Issues in Law and Medicine* 17 (2002): 229, 247, 227.

141. Keown, *Euthanasia, Ethics and Public Policy*, pp. 90, 147, 148.

142. Although some of these data became available after the two critics put forth their harsh criticism, there is no indication that either Hendin or Keown have been swayed by these new data or that they have abandoned their principled opposition to euthanasia and PAS.

143. Onwuteaka-Philipsen et al. (May 22, 2007). Available at http://www.minvws. nl/themes/euthanasia (pp. 15, 17); accessed January 17, 2010.

144. Ibid., p. 16.

145. Have, "End-of-Life Decision Making in the Netherlands," in Blank and Merrick, eds. *End-of-Life Decision Making*, p. 151.

146. Onwuteaka-Philipsen et al. (May 22, 2007). Available at http://www.minvws. nl/themes/euthanasia (p. 16); accessed January 17, 2010.

147. G.A.M. Widdershoven, "Euthanasia in the Netherlands: Experience in a Review Committtee," *Medicine and Law* 23 (2004): 691.

148. Neil M. Gorsuch, *The Future of Assisted Suicide and Euthanasia* (Princeton, NJ: Princeton University Press, 2006), p. 110.

149. Griffiths et al., *Euthanasia and Law*, p. 155.

150. Rietjens et al., "Using Drugs to End Life Without an Explicit Request of the Patient," p. 208.

151. In addition to the Rietjens study, see, e.g., Agnes van der Heide "End-of Life Decision-making in Six European Countries: Descriptive Study," *The Lancet* 362 (2003): 345–50.

152. John Griffiths et al., *Euthanasia and Law in Europe* (Oxford: Hart, 2008), p. 520.

153. Raphael Cohen-Almagor, *The Right to Die with Dignity: An Argument in Ethics, Medicine and Law* (New Brunswick, NJ: Rutgers University Press, 2001), p. 155. Cohen-Almagor, a one-time supporter of euthanasia, after a study visit to the Netherlands in 1999, is now an opponent of the Dutch regime.

154. Cohen-Almagor, *The Right to Die with Dignity* reproduces letters by Dutch scholars who assert that there exists a lively debate on end-of-life issues.

155. Griffiths et al., *Euthanasia and Law*, p. 28.

156. Thomasma et al., *Asking to Die*, p. 263.

157. Ibid., pp. 310, 298, 313.

158. Ibid., pp. 332, 340, 291.

159. Ibid., pp. 306–07.

160. Ilinka Haverkate et al., "The Emotional Impact on Physicians of Hastening the Death of a Patient," *Medical Journal of Australia* 175 (2001): 520–22.

161. Guy A.M. Widdershoven, "Beyond Autonomy and Beneficence: The Moral Basis of Euthanasia in the Netherlands," in Schotsmans and Meulenberg, eds., *Euthanasia and Palliative Care in the Low Countries*, p. 91.

Chapter 3

1. John Griffiths et al., *Euthanasia and Law in Europe* (Oxford and Portland, OR: Hart Publishing, 2008), pp. 276–79.

2. Johan Bilsen, *End-of-Life Decisions in Medical Practice in Flanders, Belgium* (Brussels: Free University of Brussels, 2005), p. 44.

3. Margo Trappenburg and Joop van Holsteyn, "The Quest for Limits: Law and Public Opinion on Euthanasia in the Netherlands," in *Regulating Physician-Negotiated Death,* edited by Albert Klijn et al. (s'Gravenhage: Elsevier, 2001), p. 143

4. Bilsen, *End-of-Life Decisions in Medical Practice in Flanders,* p. 76.

5. Ibid., p. 50. See also Johan Bilsen et al., "The Incidence and Characteristics of End-of-Life Decisions by GPs in Belgium," *Family Practice* 21 (2004): 286.

6. Luc Deliens et al., "End-of-Life Decisions in Medical Practice in Flanders, Belgium: A Nationwide Study," *The Lancet* 356 (2000): 1811.

7. Bilsen, *End-of-Life Decisions in Medical Practice in Flanders,* p. 54.

8. Ibid., p. 139. This study was also published as "Involvement of Nurses in Physician-assisted Dying," *Journal of Advanced Nursing* 47 (2004): 583–91.

9. Bilsen, *End-of-Life Decisions in Medical Practice in Flanders,* pp. 84, 90–91.

10. Luc Deliens and Freddy Mortier, "Empirical Research on End-of-Life Decisions in Medical Practice in Belgium (Flanders)," in *Clinical and Epidemiological Aspects of End-of-Life Decision-Making,* edited by Agnes van der Heide et al. (Amsterdam: Royal Dutch Academy of Arts and Sciences, 2001), p.122.

11. Joachim Cohen, *End-of-Life Decisions and Place of Death in Belgium and Europe* (Brussels: Brussels University Press, 2007), p. 39.

12. Griffiths et al., *Euthanasia and Law in Europe,* pp. 279–80.

13. Bert Broeckaert, "Towards a Legal Recognition of Euthanasia," *European Journal of Health Law* 8 (2001): 95–96.

14. Ibid., pp. 96–98; Griffiths et al., *Euthanasia and Law in Europe,* pp. 280–81.

15. Bert Broeckaert, "Towards a Legal Recognition of Euthanasia," pp. 101–103; Maurice Adams, "Euthanasia: The Process of Legal Change in Belgium – Reflections on the Parliamentary Debate," in *Regulating Physician-Negotiated Death,* edited by Albert Klijn et al. (s'Gravenhage: Elsevier, 2001), pp. 40–43.

16. Ibid., p. 47; Griffiths et al., *Euthanasia and Law in Europe,* pp. 289–291.

17. *Belgish Staatsblad,* June 22, 2002. For an English translation see "The Belgian Act on Euthanasia of May 28, 2002," *Ethical Perspectives* 9 (2002): 182–88. The same translation, supervised by Prof. Herman Nys of the Center for Biomedical Ethics and Law at the Catholic University of Leuven, is used in Appendix 1 of *Euthanasia and Palliative Care in the Low Countries,* edited by Paul Schotmans and Tom Meulenbergs (Leuven: Peeters, 2005), and is reprinted in Appendix 2 of the present work (pp. 172–81).

18. Commission Fédérale de Contrôle et d'Evaluation de l'Euthanasie, *Brochure à l'Intention du Corps Médicale,* appendix to *Deuxième Rapport aux Chambres Législatives* (Brussels, 2006). Available at www.health.fgov.be/agp/fr/eutha-nasie/f5764rapporteuthanasiefr.pdf.

19. Luc Deliens et al., "Similitudes et Différences entre les Lois Belge et Néérlandaise relatives à l'Euthanasie," *Revue Médicale de Liège* 58 (2003): 487.

20. Griffiths et al., *Euthanasia and Law in Europe*, pp. 310–11.
21. Commission Fédérale de Contrôle et d'Evaluation de l'Euthanasie, *Brochure à l'Intention du Corps Médicale*, sect. 7.
22. Griffiths et al., *Euthanasia and Law in Europe*, p. 311.
23. Maurice Adams and Herman Nys, "Euthanasia in the Low Countries: Comparative Reflections on the Belgian and Dutch Euthanasia Act," in *Euthanasia and Palliative Care in the Low Countries*, edited by Schotmans and Meulenbergs, pp. 8–9.
24. *Belgish Staatsblad*, June 14, 2002. The law is summarized in the International Digest of Health Legislation published by the World Health Organization, Belg.04.002. Available at www.who.int/idhl.
25. Commission Fédérale de Contrôle et d'Evaluation de l'Euthanasie, *Brochure à l'Intention du Corps Médicale*, sect. 3.
26. *Belgish Staatsblad*, December 13, 2005; Griffiths et al., *Euthanasia and Law in Europe*, p. 322.
27. The reports can be found on line. For the URL see n. 18 above.
28. Griffiths et al., *Euthanasia and Law in Europe*, p. 337.
29. Marc Englert, "Deux années d'euthanasie dépénalisee en Belgique: Comparasion avec les Pays-Bas. Premier bilan d'une unite de soins palliatifs," *Revue médicale de Bruxelles* 26 (2005): 150.
30. Lieve van den Block, *End-of-Life Care and Medical Decision-Making in the Last Phase of Life* (Brussels: Brussels University Press, 2008), p. 151.
31. Lieve Van den Block et al., "Euthanasia and Other Life-ending Decisions: A Mortality Follow-back Study in Belgium," *BMC Public Health* 9 (2009): 84.
32. Griffiths et al., *Euthanasia and Law in Europe*, p. 343.
33. Ibid., pp. 341–42.
34. Agnes van der Heide, "End-of-Life Decision-making in Six European Countries: Descriptive Study," *The Lancet* 361 (2003): 347.
35. Commission Fédérale de Contrôle et d'Evaluation de l'Euthanasie., *Troisième Rapport aux Chambres Législatives* (Brussels, 2008), pp. 21–22.
36. Joachim Cohen et al., "Influence of Physicians' Life Stances on Attitudes to End-of-Life Decisions and Actual End-of-Life Decision-making in Six Countries," *Journal of Medical Ethics* 4 (2008): 251.
37. Freddy Mortier and Luc Deliens, "The Prospects of Legal Control on Euthanasia in Belgium: Implications of Recent End-of-Life Studies," in *Regulating Physician-Negotiated Death*, edited by Albert Klijn et al. (s'Gravenhage: Elsevier, 2001), p. 182.
38. Georg Bosshard et al., "A Role for Doctors in Assisted Dying? An Analysis of Legal Regulations and Medical Professional Positions in Six European Countries," *Journal of Medical Ethics* 34 (2008):29–30.

39. The statement of December 4, 2003 and related matters can be found at www.consciencelaws.org.
40. Griffiths et al., *Euthanasia and Law in Europe*, pp. 321–22.
41. C. Gastmans et al., "Facing Requests for Euthanasia: A Clinical Practice Guideline," *Journal of Medical Ethics* 30 (2004): 212–13.
42 According to data provided by Joke Lemiengre et al., "Ethics Policies on Euthanasia in Nursing Homes: A Survey in Flanders, Belgium," *Social Science and Medicine* 66 (2008): 383, most nursing homes affiliated with Caritas (86%) permit euthanasia for competent, terminally ill patients according to the Caritas guidelines, 4% according to the law, and 10% do not permit it at all.
43. Ibid., pp. 213–15.
44. Jan Jans, "Churches in the Low Countries on Euthanasia: Background, Argumentation and Commentary," in "Palliative Care and Euthanasia: Belgian and Dutch Perspectives," in *Euthanasia and Palliative Care in the Low Countries*, pp. 186–89.
45. Chris Gastmans et al., "Pluralism and Ethical Dialogue in Christian Health care Institutions: The View of Caritas Catholica Flanders," *Christian Bioethics* 12 (2006): 271–78.
46. Englert, "Deux années d'euthanasie dépénalisee en Belgique," p. 148.
47. "Hugo Claus," Wikipedia.
48. Bert Broeckaert and Rien Janssens, "Palliative Care and Euthanasia: Belgian and Dutch Perspectives," in *Euthanasia and Palliative Care in the Low Countries*, pp. 44–46. See also the FPZV statement "Decisions on the Border Between Life and Death" of September 6, 2003. Available at www.consciencelaws.org; accessed January 20, 2010.
49. Broeckaert and Janssens, "Palliative Care and Euthanasia," pp. 47–54.
50. C. Gastmans et al., "Facing Requests for Euthanasia: A Clinical Practice Guideline," *Journal of Medical Ethics* 30 (2004): 216.
51. Jan Bernheim et al., "Development of Palliative Care and Legalization of Euthanasia: Antagonism or Synergy?" *British Medical Journal* 336 (2008): 864.
52. Caroline Buisseret et al., "Palliative Care Associations: The Belgian experience," *European Journal of Palliative Care* 10 (2003): 247–49. See also the 2005 report of the European Task Force on Palliative Care (EAPC) in *European Journal of Palliative Care* 13 (2006), no. 4.
53. Bernheim et al., "Development of Palliative Care and Legalization of Euthanasia," p. 864.
54. Lieve Van den Block, "Care for Patients in the Last Months of Life: The Belgian Sentinel Network Monitoring End-of-Life Care Study," *Archives of Internal Medicine* 168 (2008): 1751.
55. Englert, "Deux années d'euthanasie dépénalisee en Belgique," p. 151.

56. Van den Block, *End-of-Life Care and Medical Decision-Making in the Last Phase of Life*, pp. 170–71. This study will also be published in 2009 as Lieve Van den Block et al., "How Are Euthanasia and Other End-of-Life Decisions Related to the Care Provided in the Final Three Months of Life? A Nationwide Mortality Follow-back Study in Belgium," in the *British Medical Journal.*

Chapter 4

1. Olivier Guillod and Aline Schmidt, "Assisted Suicide Under Swiss Law," *European Journal of Health Law* 12 (2005): 25. For the full text of these provisions see Appendix 3 of this work (p. 182).
2. Agnes van der Heide et al., "End-of-life decision making in six European countries: descriptive study," *The Lancet* 361 (2003): 347.
3. Bundesamt für Justiz, Report "Sterbehilfe und Palliativmedizin – Handlungsbedarf für den Bund?" Bern, April 24, 2006. Available at www.bj.admin.ch/bj/de/home/themen/gesellschaft/gesetzgebung/sterbehilfe.html; accessed January 21, 2010.
4. "Ergänzung des Freitodbegleiterteams," Exit Bulletin no. 59 (1997), p. 20.
5. Gabriele Fricker, *Aus freiem Willen, Der Tod als Erlösung: Erfahrungen einer Freitodbegleiterin* (Zurich: Oesch, 1999), p. 44; "Exit by <Exit>: Geschäftsführer Holenstein abgewählt," *Neue Zürcher Zeitung,* May 18, 1998.
6. "Die Regierung zu den Aktivitäten von <Exit>: Strafverfahren gegen Professor Schär hängig," *Neue Zürcher Zeitung,* July 9, 1999.
7. "Exit-Präsident Rudolf Syz zurückgetreten," *Neue Zürcher Zeitung,* May 17, 1999.
8. Fricker, *Aus freiem* Willen, pp. 34–35; Exit info (1/2008), p. 6.
9. An edited version of this opinion was published as Klaus Peter Rippe et al.,"Urteilsfähigkeit von Menschen mit psychischen Störungen und Suizidbeihilfe," *Schweizerische Juristen-Zeitung* 101 (2005): 53–62, 81–91.
10. Exit, *Selbstbestimmung im Leben und im Sterben* (June 2005), p. 14.
11. BGE 133 I 58, p. 75. Available at www.bger.ch.
12. "Exit-Spitze macht gute Geschäfte mit dem Tod," *Schweizer Beobachter* (Glattburg), March 16, 2001.
13. "Nebengeräusche statt Inhalt: Vor der Exit-Generalversammlung," *Neue Zürcher Zeitung,* May 19, 2001.
14. *Tages-Anzeiger,* November 15, 2007.
15. Ibid.
16. *Sonntagsblick,* November 21, 2007.
17. Georg Bosshard et al., "748 Cases of Suicide Assisted by a Swiss Right-to-Die Organization," *Swiss Medical Weekly* 133 (2003): 316.

18. Exit, *Selbstbestimmung im Leben und im Sterben*, pp. 9–10.
19. Exit info (1/2008), p. 14.
20. Ibid., and Exit, *Selbstbestimmung im Leben und im Sterben*, pp. 11–14.
21. Susanne Fischer et al., "Suicide Assisted by Two Swiss Right-to-Die Organizations," *Journal of Medical Ethics* 34 (2008): 812–13.
22. Stephen Ziegler and George Bosshard, "Role of Non-Governmental Organizations in Physician Assisted Suicide," *British Medical Journal* 334 (2007): 296.
23. Svenja Flasspöhler, *Mein Wille Geschehe: Sterben in Zeiten der Freitodhilfe* (Berlin: WJS, 2007), pp. 44–45. See also Fricker, *Aus freiem* Willen, p. 44.
24. Exit info (1/2008), p. 15.
25. Ibid.
26. Undated Exit report, distributed by ERGO (Euthanasia Research and Guidance Organization), Junction City, OR, under the date of August 2, 2001. Available at www.finalexit.org/swissframe.html.
27. Flasspöhler, *Mein Wille Geschehe*, p. 57.
28. Interview with Exit official Heidi Vogt Daeneker, Leiterin Freitodbegleitung, July 9, 2008.
29. Bosshard et al., "748 Cases of Suicide Assisted by a Swiss Right-to-Die Organization," pp. 312–13. The study did not collect information relevant to the medico-legal investigation (diagnosis, etc.) for all of the 748 cases of assisted suicide carried out by Exit during 1990–2000. Hence, the percentage of nonterminal cases is known only for Canton Zurich.
30. Fischer et al., "Suicide Assisted by Two Swiss Right-to-Die Organizations," p. 812.
31. Exit, *Selbstbestimmung im Leben und im Sterben*, p. 16.
32. Ibid., p. 6.
33. Bosshard et al., "748 Cases of Suicide Assisted by a Swiss Right-to-Die Organization," p. 316.
34. Exit info (1/2008), p. 30.
35. "Sterbehilfeorganisationen suchen Psychiater: Hohe Hürden für Suizidhilfe bei psychisch kranken Menschen," *Neue Zürcher Zeitung*, June 23, 2007.
36. Exit info (1/2008), p. 18.
37. "Sterbehilfeorganisationen suchen Psychiater," p. 2.
38. Georg Bosshard et al., "Assessment of Requests for Assisted Suicide by a Swiss Right-to-Die Organization," *Death Studies* 32 (2008): 650, 653–56.
39. Andreas Frei et al., "Beihilfe zum Suizid bei psychisch Kranken," *Nervenarzt* 70 (1999): 1018; Andreas Frei et al., "Assisted Suicide as conducted by a "Right-to-Die" Society in Switzerland: A Descriptive Analysis of 43 Cases," *Swiss Medical Weekly* 131 (2001): 378–79.

40. Rippe et al.,"Urteilsfähigkeit von Menschen mit psychischen Störungen und Suizidbeihilfe," p. 91; Peter Holenstein, "Letzte Hilfe," *Weltwoche*, no. 34 (2004). Available at www.weltwoche.ch; accessed January 21, 2010.

41. Exit info (1/2008), p. 17; interview with Exit official Heidi Vogt Daeneker, Leiterin Freitodbegleitung, July 9, 2008.

42. J. Strnad et al., "Suizid in der stationären Psychiatrie unter Beihilfe einer Sterbehilfevereinigung: Fälle aktiver Sterbehilfe?" *Nervenarzt* 70 (1999): 645–49.

43. Exit info (1/2008), p. 17.

44. Bosshard et al., "748 Cases of Suicide Assisted by a Swiss Right-to-Die Organization," p. 314.

45. Flasspöhler, *Mein Wille Geschehe*, p. 85.

46. Bundesamt für Justiz, Report "Sterbehilfe und Palliativmedizin – Handlungsbedarf für den Bund?" Bern, April 24, 2006, p. 36, n. 82.

47. Ibid.

48. Fischer et al., "Suicide Assisted by Two Swiss Right-to-Die Organizations," p. 812.

49. Ibid., pp. 315–16.

50. Flasspöhler, *Mein Wille Geschehe*, p. 147.

51. Fischer et al., "Suicide Assisted by Two Swiss Right-to-Die Organizations," p. 812.

52. "Zustimmung zur Suizid-Beihilfe in Heimen," *Neue Zürcher Zeitung*, February 8, 2001.

53. Exit info (1/2008), pp. 16–17.

54. Fischer et al., "Suicide Assisted by Two Swiss Right-to-Die Organizations," p. 812.

55. Michael Meier, "Sterbehilfe via Plastiksack verurteilt," *Tages-Anzeiger*, December 29, 2000; "Erstmals eine Gefängnisstrafe," *Freiburger Nachrichten*, January 11, 2001.

56. Bosshard et al., "748 Cases of Suicide Assisted by a Swiss Right-to-Die Organization," pp. 314–15.

57. Georg Bosshard, "Switzerland," in John Griffiths et al., *Euthanasia and Law in Europe* (Oxford: Hart, 2008), p. 475.

58. Exit, *Selbstbestimmung im Leben und im Sterben* (June 2005), p. 8.

59. Interview on July 10, 2008.

60. Bosshard et al., "748 Cases of Suicide Assisted by a Swiss Right-to-Die Organization," p. 315.

61. "Vereinbarung über die organisierte Suizidhilfe," between Ober staats anwalt schaft des Kantons Zurich and Exit Deutsche Schweiz.

62. *A.D.M.D. Bulletin*, no. 49 (2008), p. 6.

63. Sandra Burkhardt et al., "L'assistance au suicide en Suisse romande: une étude sur cinq ans," *Journal de Médicine Légale Droit Médicale*, vol. 50, no. 1–2 (2007): 43.

64. Burkhardt et al., "L'assistance au suicide en Suisse romande," p. 42.

65. Maryam Zaré et al., "L'assistance au suicide en Suisse dans la contexte de polypathologie invalidante irréversible," *Revue Médicale Suisse*, no. 128 (October 10, 2007): 2303–2305.

66. *A.D.M.D. Bulletin*, no. 49 (2008), p. 14.

67. Burkhardt et al., "L'assistance au suicide en Suisse romande," p. 43.

68. J. Pereira et al., "The Response of a Swiss University Hospital's Palliative Care Consult Team to Assisted Suicide Within the Institution," *Palliative Medicine* 22 (2008): 660–63.

69. Ibid., p. 661.

70. At www.dignitas.ch. (By 2008, this website was no longer active.)

71. Available at www.lemonde/archive; "Dignitas (Verein)," Wikipedia 2007.

72. Fischer et al., "Suicide Assisted by Two Swiss Right-to-Die Organizations," p. 812.

73. "Dignitas Gründer wehrt sich," *Neue Zürcher Zeitung*, January 22, 2007.

74. Fischer et al., "Suicide Assisted by Two Swiss Right-to-Die Organizations," p. 812.

75. Peter Holenstein, "Leichen als Geiseln (interview with Ludwig Minelli)," *Weltwoche*, April 22, 2004.

76. Ludger Fittkau, "Das Reisebüro für Lebensmüde," *Frankfurter Allgemeine Zeitung* on line (FAZ.NET), March 3, 2008.

77. Available at www.dignitas.ch, report for the year 2004, p. 15; "Suicide-Clinic Entrepreneur: Depressed? We Never Say No," Minelli interview with the London *Sunday Times*, World Net Daily, April 16, 2006.

78. Alexandra Williams, "Assisted Suicide in Apartment Irks Residents," *London Sunday Telegraph*, June 10, 2006.

79. "Dignitas im Gegenwind," NZZ Online, September 28, 2007; "Wohnung der Dignitas in Stäfa geschlossen," ibid., September 27, 2007; "Weitere Gemeinde verbietet Verein Dignitas Sterbehilfe," ibid., September 28, 2007; "Dignitas sorgt für Empörung," Swissinfo, November 8, 2007.

80. Interview with Claude Fuchs, secretary, Schweizerische Gesellschaft für palliative Medizin, July 9, 2008; *Neue Zürcher Zeitung*, March 26, 2008.

81. Urs Willmann, "Dignitas ist ein diktatorischer Verein," *Die Zeit*, no. 44, October 27, 2005.

82. "Minelli verspricht Transparenz," *Basler Zeitung*, July 7, 2008.

83. "Zürcher Ermittlungen gegen Sterbehilfeorganisation Dignitas," Swissinfo, March 22, 2007; "Zürcher Kantonsrat ganz knapp gegen Verbot von Sterbetourismus," ibid., October 29, 2007.

84. Peter Baumann, "Beihilfe zum Suizid kann eine ärztliche Handlung sein," *Schweizerische Ärztezeitung* 82 (2001): 296–98; "Suizidhilfe," Available at www. suizidhilfe.ch.; accessed January 21, 2010; "Peter Baumann (Psychiater)." Available at http://de.wikipedia.org/wiki/Peter_Baumann_(Psychiater); accessed January 21, 2010.

85. Georg Bosshard, "Die Tätigkeit der Sterbehilfsorganisationen und die Rolle des Arztes," in *Beihilfe zum Suizid in der Schweiz: Beiträge aus Ethik, Recht und Medizin*, edited by Christoph Rehmann-Sutter (Bern: Peter Lang, 2008), p. 476.

86. "Sterbehelfer Baumann verurteilt," NZZ Online, July 6, 2007; Swissinfo, October 1, 2008.

87. Peter Baumann, *Suizid und Suizidhilfe: Eine Neue Sicht* (Norderstedt: Books on Demand, 2007).

88. Exit info (1/2008), p. 33.

89. "Dignitas Wirbel schadet Berner Sterbehilfe," *Tages Anzeiger*, October 8, 2007; "Sterberaum gesucht," available at www.espace.ch; accessed May 23, 2008.

90. Available at www.geocities.com/friends_at_the_end/ex-international-weibel-luxembourg2006.html.

91. See *Neue Zurcher Zeitung* of April 29, 1998, November 5, 1998, and December 22, 1999.

92. Samia A. Hurst and Alex Mauron, "Assisted Suicide and Euthanasia in Switzerland: Allowing a Role for Non-physicians," *British Medical Journal* 326 (2003): 272.

93. "Schweizer für Sterbehilfe und gegen Sterbetourismus," Swissinfo, October 7, 2007.

94. *Neue Zürcher Zeitung*, August 28, 2008.

95. Susanne Fischer et al., "Swiss Doctors' Attitudes Towards End-of-Life Decisions and Their Determinants: A Comparison of Three Language Regions," *Swiss Medical Weekly* 135 (2005): 373.

96. Sandra Burkhardt et al., "Assistance au suicide en Suisse: La position des médecins," *Revue Médicale Suisse*, no. 137 (December 12, 2007): 2862.

97. The full report can be read at www.bj.admin.ch. See also Olivier Guillod and Aline Schmidt, "Assisted Suicide Under Swiss Law," *European Journal of Health Law* 12 (2005):32–33.

98. Cf. Georg Bosshard and Walter Bär, "Sterbeassistenz und die Rolle des Arztes," *Aktuelle Juristische Praxis* 11 (2002): 409–13.

99. Guillod and Schmidt, "Assisted Suicide Under Swiss Law," pp. 33–34.

100. Swiss Academy of Medical Sciences (SAMW), "Betreuung von Patienten am Lebensende: Medizinisch-ethische Richtlinien der SAMS," November 25, 2004.

101. The report is available in German, French, Italian, and English, and can be read at www.nek-cne.ch. The text quoted is on p. 62 of the English version.
102. Ibid., pp. 64, 66.
103. Ibid., p. 65.
104. Ibid., p. 67.
105. Ibid., p. 68.
106. Ibid., p. 69.
107. Ibid., p. 70.
108. Ibid., p. 71.
109. Ibid., p. 72.
110. Ibid., p.73.
111. National Advisory Commission on Biomedical Ethics, "Duty-of-Care Criteria for the Management of Assisted Suicide," Opinion No. 13/2006.
112. Ibid., pp. 4–6.
113. N. Bittel et al., "'Euthanasia': A Survey by the Swiss Association for Palliative Care," *Supportive Care in Cancer* 10 (2002): 265–71.
114. Available at www.palliative.ch.
115. National Advisory Commission on Biomedical Ethics, Opinion No. 9/2005, pp. 9, 36.
116. Ruth Baumann-Hölzle, "Der Tod als Freund," *Schweizerische Ärztezeitung* 84 (2003): 2427.
117. Georg Bosshard, "Die Tätigkeit der Sterbehilfeorganisationen und die Rolle des Arztes," in *Beihilfe zum Suizid in der Schweiz*, edited by Rehmann-Sutter et al., p. 30.
118. *Neue Zürcher Zeitung*, November 12/13, 2005, cited by Eidgenössisches Justiz- und Polizeidepartement (EJPD), "Sterbehilfe und Palliativmedizin – Handlungsbedarf für den Bund?" draft of January 31, 2006 (which appears to be identical with the final version released on April 24, 2006), p. 17. The document can be read on the website of the Federal Department of Justice and Police, at www.ejpd.admin.ch.
119. Ibid., pp. 43, 45.
120. Ibid., p. 46.
121. Ibid., p. 52.
122. EJPD, "Ergänzungsbericht zum Bericht 'Sterbehilfe und Palliativmedizin – Handlungsbedarf für den Bund?'" July 2007, pp. 6–8.
123. Ibid., pp. 9–11.
124. "Sterbehilfe gibt weiterhin zu redden," Swissinfo, June 1, 2006.
125. "Nur die wenigsten haben eine Patientenverfügung," *Tages Anzeiger*, January 21, 2008.
126. NZZ Online, June 13, 2007.

127. "Zürcher Kantonsrat ganz knapp gegen Verbot von Sterbetourismus, "Swissinfo, October 29, 2007.
128. EJPD, "Ergänzungsbericht zum Bericht 'Sterbehilfe und Palliativmedizin," July 2007, p. 2/12, n. 1.
129. BGE 133 I 58, p. 75. Available at www.bger.ch.
130. "Widmer-Schlumpf will professionelle Betreuung von Sterbewilligen," Swissinfo, July 13, 2008.
131. "Kantonsinitiative gegen Sterbetourismus," ibid., June 17, 2008.
132. "Bundesrat macht Wende bei Sterbehilfe," ibid., July 2, 2008.
133. News release of Ministry of Justice, October 28, 2009.
134. Swissinfo, October 31, 2009.

Chapter 5

1. Katherine Ann Wingfield and Carl S. Hacker, "Physician-Assisted Suicide: An Assessment and Comparison of Statutory Approaches Among the States," *Seton Hall Legislative Journal* 32 (2007): 56.
2. *Washington v. Glucksberg,* 521 U.S. 702 (1997) and *Vacco v. Quill,* 521 U.S. 193 (1997).
3. *Lee v. Oregon,* 891 F. Supp. 1429 (D.Or. 1995).
4. *Lee v. Oregon,* 107 F. 3 1382 (9 Circ. 1997).
5. For more detail, see Susan M. Behuniak and Arthur G. Svenson, *Physician-assisted Suicide: The Anatomy of Constitutional Law Issue* (Lanham, MD: Rowman and Littlefield, 2003), p. 83.
6. Susan E. Hickman, "Physicians' and Nurses' Perspectives on Increased Family Reports of Pain in Dying Hospitalized Patients," *Journal of Palliative Medicine* 3 (2000): 414–17.
7. Ibid., p. 176; Margaret P. Pattin, "New Life in the Assisted-Death Debate in the United States: Scheduled Drugs v. NuTech," in *Regulating Physician-Negotiated Death,* edited by Albert Klijn et al., pp. 54–55.
8. The text of this ruling is reprinted in *Issues in Law and Medicine* 17 (2002): 269–92.
9. *Gonzales v. Oregon,* 546 U.S. 243 (2006).
10. Tony Farrenkopf and James Bryan, "Psychological Consultation Under Oregon's 1994 Death with Dignity Act: Ethics and Procedures," *Professional Psychology: Research and Practice* 30 (1999):247.
11. Oregon Revised Statutes (1997), Chapter 127.800–127.897. The text of the law can also be found on the Oregon Department of Human Services' Death with Dignity website. It is reprinted in Margaret P. Battin et al., eds., *Physician-assisted*

Suicide: Expanding the Debate (New York: Routledge, 1998), Appendix D, pp. 443–48, and in this work in Appendix 4 (pp. 183–97).

12. Oregon Administrative Rules 333–009–000 to 333–009–0030. Available at http://egov.oregon.gov/DHS/ph/pas/oars.shtml. See also Katrina Hedberg and Susan W. Tolle, "Physician-assisted Suicide in Care of Dying: The Oregon Perspective," in *Assisted Suicide: Finding Common Ground,* edited by Lois Snyder and Arthur L. Kaplan (Bloomington: Indiana University Press, 2002), pp. 10–11.

13. "FAQ About the Death with Dignity Act," to be found under the Oregon Department of Human Services' Death with Dignity website.

14. Cf. Barbara Coombs Lee, "Physician-assisted Suicide," in *Oregon Health Law Manual,* vol. 2: *Life and Death Decisions* (Lake Oswego: Oregon State Bar, 1997), pp. 8–19. See also Linda Ganzini et al., "Attitudes of Patients with Amyotrophic Lateral Sclerosis and Their Caregivers Toward Assisted Suicide," *New England Journal of Medicine* 339 (1998): 971.

15. Communication from Dr. Katrina Hedberg, Oregon Public Health Division, November 5, 2007.

16. Task Force to Improve the Care of Terminally Ill Oregonians, *The Oregon Death with Dignity Act: A Guidebook for Health Care Professionals* (Oregon Health and Science University, 2007), p. 55.

17. For the 2008 summary report and other yearly reports of the Oregon Department of Human Services, see the Department of Human Services' Death with Dignity website. Available at http://oregon.gov/DHS/ph/pas/index.shtml.

18. Susan W. Tolle, et al., "Characteristics and Proportion of Dying Oregonians who Personally Consider Physician-assisted Suicide," *Journal of Clinical Ethics* 15 (2004): 113–14.

19. These figures are taken from the Tenth Annual Report on Oregon's Death with Dignity Act. See also Howard Wineberg and James L. Werth, "Physician-assisted Suicide in Oregon: What Are the Key Factors?" *Death Studies* 27 (2003): 510–11.

20. Ibid., pp. 505–507.

21. Ibid., pp. 509–10; Linda Ganzini et al., "Oregon Physicians' Perceptions of Patients Who Request Assisted Suicide and Their Families," *Journal of Palliative Medicine* 6 (2003): 382–83, 389; Bryant Carlson et al., "Oregon Hospice Chaplains' Experience with Patients Requesting Physician-assisted Suicide," *Journal of Palliative Medicine* 8 (2005): 1165; Linda Ganzini et al., "Experiences of Oregon Nurses and Social Workers with Hospice Patients Who Requested Assistance with Suicide," *New England Journal of Medicine* 347 (2002): 584; Tolle et al., "Characteristics and Proportion of Dying Oregonians," pp. 114–15.

22. Ganzini et al., "Experiences of Oregon Nurses and Social Workers with Hospice Patients Who Requested Assistance with Suicide," p. 585.

23. Oregon Department of Human Services, 2008 Summary of Oregon's Death with Dignity Act (March, 2009).

24. Wineberg and Werth, "Physician-assisted Suicide in Oregon," p. 511; Oregon Hospice Association, Summary Report for 2004 (June 18, 2005). Available at www.oregonhospice.org.

25. Oregon Hospice Association, Annual report for 2006 (January 26, 2007); Ann Jackson, "Hospice in Oregon 2008: A Historical Perspective," March 4, 2008, ibid.

26. Statement with regard to *Gonzales v. Oregon* (2006), ibid.

27. Linda Ganzini et al., "Oregon Physicians' Attitudes About and Experiences with End-of-Life Care Since Passage of the Oregon Death with Dignity Act," *Journal of the American Medical Association* 285 (2001): 2365.

28. Steven Dobscha, "Oregon Physicians' Responses to Requests for Assisted Suicide: A Qualitative Study," *Journal fof Palliative Medicine* 7 (2004): 451–61.

29. Arthur E. Chin, "Legalized Physician-assisted Suicide in Oregon: The First Year's Excperience," *New England Journal of Medicine* 340 (1999): 583.

30. Linda Ganzini et al., "Physicians' Experiences with the Oregon Death with Dignity Act," *New England Journal of Medicine* 342 (2000): 561.

31. Ganzini et al., "Oregon Physicians' Attitudes About and Experiences with End-of-Life Care," p. 2368.

32. Lois L. Miller, "Attitudes and Experiences of Oregon Hospice Nurses and Social Workers Regarding Assisted Suicide," *Palliative Medicine* 18 (2004):687–89. For a study with similar results, see Ganzini et al., "Experiences of Oregon Nurses and Social Workers with Hospice Patients Who Requested Assistance with Suicide," pp. 582–88.

33. Kristine Carlson Marcus, "Pharmacists's Response to Oregon's Death with Dignity Act," in *Drug Use in Assisted Suicide and Euthanasia*, edited by Margaret P. Battin and Arthur G. Lipman (New York: Haworth Press, 1996), p. 155.

34. Frank Baumeister and Patricia Dunn, "Attending Physician and Consulting Physician," in *The Death with Dignity Act: A Guidebook for Health Care Providers*, edited by Task Force to Improve the Care of the Terminally Ill Oregonians (Portland: Oregon Health Sciences University, 1998), p. 25. The same language appears in the 2008 edition of the Guidebook.

35. Linda Ganzini et al., "Prevalence of Depression and Anxiety in Patients Requesting Physicians' Aid in Dying: Cross-sectional Survey," *British Medical Journal* 337 (2008): 973.

36. Raphael Cohen-Almagor, *The Right to Die with Dignity: An Argument in Ethics, Medicine and Law* (New Brunswick, NJ: Rutgers University Press, 2001), p. 133.

37. Sherwin B. Nuland, "Physician-assisted Suicide and Euthanasia in Practice," *New England Journal of Medicine* 342 (2000): 584.

38. *The Oregon Death with Dignity Act: A Guidebook for Health Care Professionals* (2007 edition), p. 20. See also Terri A. Schmidt et al., "The Physician Orders for Life-sustaining Treatment [POLST] Program: Oregon Emergency Medical Technicianss Practical Experiences and Attitudes," *Journal of the American Geriatric Society* 52 (2007): 1430–1434.

39. Amy D. Sullivan et al., "Legalized Physician-assisted Suicide in Oregon: The Second Year," *New England Journal of Medicine* 342 (2000): 603.

40. ORS 677.415, 441.057; *The Oregon Death with Dignity Act: A Guidebook for Health Care Professionals* (2007 edition), p. 78.

41. John Keown, *Euthanasia, Ethics and Public Policy: An Argument Against Legislation* (Cambridge: Cambridge University Press, 2002), p. 173.

42. Eric G. Campbell et al., "Professionalism in Medicine: Results of a National Survey of Physicians," *Annals of Internal Medicine* 147 (2007): 795–802.

43. Kathleen Foley and Herbert Hendin, *The Case Against Assisted Suicide: For the Right to End-of-Life Care* (Baltimore, MD: Johns Hopkins University Press, 2002), p. 159.

44. Katrina Hedberg and Karen Southwick, "Legalized Physician-assisted Suicide in Oregon, 2001," *New England Journal of Medicine* 346 (2002): 650.

45. Keown, *Euthanasia, Ethics and Public Policy*, p. 180.

46. Sullivan et al., "Legalized Physician-assisted Suicide in Oregon," p. 599.

47. Ganzini et al., "Physicians' Experiences with the Oregon Death with Dignity Act," pp. 560–61.

48. According to the *Statistical Abstract of the United States: 2004–2005*, the state of Oregon in 2002 had 8,528 non-federal physicians (Table 150, p. 107).

49. Keown, *Euthanasia, Ethics and Public Policy*, p. 179.

50. Ganzini et al., "Oregon Physicians' Attitudes About and Experiences with End-of-Life Care," p. 2368.

51. Melinda Lee and Susan W. Tolle, "Oregon's Assisted Suicide Vote: The Silver Lining," *Annals of Internal Medicine* 124 (1996): 268–69.

52. James A. Tulsky et al., "Responding to Legal Requests for Physician-assisted Suicide," *Annals of Internal Medicine* 132 (2000): 494–99.

53. Timothy E. Quill, "Legal Regulation of Physician-assisted Death: The Latest Report Card," *New England Journal of Medicine* 356 (2007): 1912.

54. See also Franklin G. Miller, "Can Physician-assisted Suicide be Regulated Effectively?" *Journal of Law, Medicine and Ethics* 24 (1996): 226–31.

55. Ezekiel J. Emanuel, "The Practice of Euthanasia and Physician-assisted Suicide in the United States: Adherence to Proposed Safeguards and Effects on Physicians," *Journal of the American Medical Association* 280 (1998): 511–12.

56. Ganzini et al., "Prevalence of Depression and Anxiety in Patients Requesting Physicians' Aid in Dying: Cross-sectional Survey," pp. 973–75.

57. L. Eisenberg, "Treating Depression and Anxiety in Primary Care: Closing the Gap Between Knowledge and Practice," *New England Journal of Medicine* 326 (1992): 1080–1084.

58. Steven D. Passik, "Oncologists' Recognition of Depression in Their Patients with Cancer," *Journal of Clinical Oncology* 16 (1998): 1597.

59. Linda Ganzini et al., "Attitudes of Oregon Psychiatrists Toward Physician-assisted Suicide," *American Journal of Psychiatry* 153 (1996): 1473.

60. Ganzini et al., "Prevalence of Depression and Anxiety in Patients Requesting Physicians' Aid in Dying: Cross-sectional Survey," p. 974–75. For a similar critical assessment, see Barry Rosenfeld, *Assisted Suicide and the Right to Die: The Interface of Social Science, Public Policy, and Medical Ethics* (Washington, DC: American Psychological Association, 2004), pp. 158–162.

61. *The Oregon Death with Dignity Act: A Guidebook for Health Care Professionals* (2007 edition), pp. 63–64.

62. Joanne M. Hilden, "Attitudes and Practices Among Pediatric Oncologists Regarding End-of-Life Care: Results of the 1998 American Society of Clinical Oncology Survey," *Journal of Clinical Oncology* 19 (2001): 208.

63. Marina Cuttini and the EURONIC Study Group, "End-of-Life Decisions in Neonatal Intensive Care: Results from a Multicenter European Study," in *Clinical and Epidemological Aspects of End-of-Life Decision-making*, edited by Agnes van der Heide et al. (Amsterdam: Royal Dutch Academy of Arts and Sciences, 2001), p. 198.

64. James Tibbals, "Legal Basis for Ethical Withholding and Withdrawing Life-sustaining Medical Treatment from Infants and Children," *Journal of Paediatrics and Child Health* 43 (2007): 235.

65. William Meadows and John Lantos, "Epidemiology and Ethics in the NICU," ibid., pp. 179–82.

66. Susan Okie, "Physician-assisted Suicide: Oregon and Beyond," *New England Journal of Medicine* 352 (2005): 1627, 1629–30.

Chapter 6

1. Paul van der Maas and Linda L. Emanuel, "Factual Findings," in *Regulating How We Die: The Ethical, Medical, and Legal Issues Surrounding Physician-assisted Suicide*, edited by Linda L. Emanuel (Cambridge, MA: Harvard University Press, 1998), p. 174.

2. Position statement on "Physician-assisted Death." Available at www.aahpm. org/positions/suicide'html.

3. Timothy Quill, "Death and Dignity: A Case of Individualized Decision Making," *New England Journal of Medicine* 324 (1991): 691–94.

4. Barry Rosenfeld, *Assisted Suicide and the Right to Die: The Interface of Social Science, Public Policy, and Medical Ethics* (Washington, DC: American Psychological Association, 2004), p. 96.

5. Neil M. Gorsuch, *The Future of Assisted Suicide and Euthanasia* (Princeton, NJ: Princeton University Press, 2006), p. 126.

6. Timothy E. Quill and Margaret E. Battin, "Excellent Palliative Care as the Standard, Physician-assisted Dying as a Last Resort," in *Physician-assisted Dying: The Case for Palliative Care and Patient Choice,* edited by Quill and Battin (Baltimore, MD: Johns Hopkins University Press, 2004), p. 330.

7. John Griffiths et al., *Euthanasia and Law in Europe* (Oxford and Portland, OR: Hart, 2008), p. 516.

8. David Orentlicher, "The Supreme Court and Physician-assisted Suicide: Rejecting Assisted Suicide but Embracing Euthanasia," *New England Journal of Medicine* 337 (1997): 1237.

9. Christian Bänziger, *Sterbehilfe für Neugeborene aus strafrechtlicher Sicht* (Zurich: Schulthess, 2006), p. 23.

10. Charles H. Baron et al., "A Model State Act to Authorize and Regulate Physician-assisted Suicide," *Harvard Journal on Legislation* 33 (1996): 1–34. The text of the model statute is on pp. 25–34. For another similar PAS regulatory scheme, see Franklin G. Miller et al., "Regulating Physician-assisted Death," *New England Journal of Medicine* 331 (1994): 119–23.

11. Baron, "A Model State Act," p. 10.

12. Ibid., p. 5.

13. Ibid., pp. 12–14.

14. Margo Trappenburg and Joop van Holsteyn, "The Quest for Limits: Law and Public Opinion on Euthanasia in the Netherlands," in *Regulating Physician-negotiated Death,* edited by Albert Klijn et al. (s'Gravenhage: Elsevier, 2001), p. 138.

15. Griffiths et al., *Euthanasia and Law in Europe,* p. 516.

16. Margaret P. Battin, *Ending Life: Ethics and the Way We Die* (New York: Oxford University Press, 2005), p. 27.

17. Margaret Otlowski, review of Magnusson, *Angels of Death,* in *Journal of Medical Ethics* 30 (2004): 2.

18. Timothy E. Quill, *A Midwife Through the Dying Process: Stories of Healing and Hard Choices at the End of Life* (Baltimore, MD: Johns Hopkins University Press, 1996), pp. 213–14.

SEEING INFECTIOUS DISEASE AS CENTRAL

Books

Bänziger, Christian. *Sterbehilfe für Neugeborene aus strafrechtlicher Sicht.* Zürich: Schulthess, 2006.

Battin, Margaret Pabst. *Ending Life: Ethics and the Way We Die.* New York: Oxford University Press, 2005.

———. *The Least Worst Death: Essays in Bioethics on the End of Life.* New York: Oxford University Press, 1994.

Battin, Margaret Pabst, et al., eds. *Physician-assisted Suicide: Expanding the Debate.* New York: Routledge, 1998.

Battin, Margaret P., and Arthur G. Lipman, eds. *Drug Use in Assisted Suicide and Euthanasia.* New York: Haworth Press, 1996.

Baumann, Peter. *Suizid und Suizidhilfe: Eine neue Sicht.* Norderstadt: Books on Demand, 2007.

Behuniak, Susan M., and Arthur G. Svenson. *Physician-assisted Suicide: The Anatomy of a Constitutional Law Issue.* Lanham, MD: Rowman and Littlefield, 2003.

Blank, Robert, and Janna C. Merrick, eds. *End-of-Life Decision Making: A Cross-National Survey.* Cambridge, MA: MIT Press, 2005.

Block, Lieve van der, et al. *End-of-Life Care and Medical Decision-making in the Last Phase of Life.* Brussels: Brussels University Press, 2008.

Cohen, Joachim. *End-of-Life Decisions and Place of Death in Belgium and Europe.* Brussels: Brussels University Press, 2007.

Cohen-Almagor, Raphael. *The Right to Die with Dignity: An Argument in Ethics, Medicine, and the Law.* New Brunswick, NJ: Rutgers University Press, 2001.

Dowbiggin, Ian. *A Merciful End: The Euthanasia Movement in Modern America.* Oxford: Oxford University Press, 2003.

Flasspöhler, Svenja. *Mein Wille Geschehe: Sterben in Zeiten der Freitodhilfe.* Berlin: WJS, 2007.

Foley, Kathleen, and Herbert Hendin. *The Case Against Assisted Suicide: For the Right to End-of-Life Care.* Baltimore, MD: Johns Hopkins University Press, 2002.

Francke, Anneke L. *Palliative Care for Terminally Ill Patients in the Netherlands.* The Hague: Ministry of Health, Welfare and Sports, 2003.

Fricker, Gabriele. *Aus freiem Willen: Der Tod als Erlösung – Erfahrungen einer Freitodbegleiterin.* Zurich: Oesch, 1999.

Gorsuch, Neil M. *The Future of Assisted Suicide and Euthanasia.* Princeton, NJ: Princeton University Press, 2006.

Griffith, John, et al. *Euthanasia and Law in Europe.* Oxford: Hart, 2008.

———. *Euthanasia and Law in the Netherlands.* Amsterdam: Amsterdam University Press, 1998.

Grundmann, Antonia. *Die niederländischen Gesetze über die Prüfung von Lebensbeendigung auf Verlangen und Beihilfe zur Selbsttötung.* Aachen: Shaker, 2004.

Have, Henk ten, and Rien Janssens, eds. *Palliative Care in Europe: Concepts and Policies.* Amsterdam: IOS Press, 2001.

Heide, Agnes van der, et al., eds. *Clinical and Epidemiological Aspects of End-of-Life Decision Making.* Amsterdam: Royal Dutch Academy of Arts and Sciences, 2001.

Hendin, Herbert. *Seduced by Death: Doctors, Patients, and the Dutch Cure.* New York: W.W. Norton, 1997.

Keown, John. *Euthanasia, Ethics and Public Policy: An Argument Against Legislation.* Cambridge: Cambridge University Press, 2002.

Klijn, Albert, et al., eds. *Regulating Physician-negotiated Death.* 's-Gravenhage: Elsevier, 2001.

Kohnen, P., and G. Schumacher, eds. *Euthanasia and Human Dignity: A Collection of Contributions by the Dutch Catholic Bishops' Conference to the Legislative Procedure 1983-2001.* Utrecht/Leuven: Peeters, 2002.

Küng, Hans, et al. *Dying with Dignity: A Plea for Personal Responsibility.* New York: Continuum, 1995.

Magnusson, Roger S. *Angels of Death: Exploring the Euthanasia Underground.* New Haven, CT: Yale University Press, 2002.

Miles, Steven M. *The Hippocratic Oath and the Ethics of Medicine.* New York: Oxford University Press, 2004.

Olick, Robert S. *Taking Advance Directives Seriously: Prospective Autonomy and Decisions near the End of Life.* Washington, DC: Georgetown University Press, 2001.

Onwuteaka-Philipsen, B.D., et al. *Evaluatie: Wet Toetsing Levensbeeindiging op Verzogek en Hulp bij Zelfdoding* (Evaluation: Act on the Termination of Life on Request and Assisted Suicide). The Hague: ZonMw, 2007.

Otlowski, Margaret. *Voluntary Euthanasia and the Common Law.* Oxford: Clarendon Press, 1997.

Pool, Robert. *Negotiating a Good Death: Euthanasia in the Netherlands.* New York: Haworth Press, 2000.

Quill, Timothy. *A Midwife Through the Dying Process: Stories of Healing and Hard Choices at the End of Life.* Baltimore, MD: Johns Hopkins University Press, 1996.

Quill, Timothy, and Margaret Battin, eds. *Physician-assisted Dying: The Case for Palliative Care and Patient Choice.* Baltimore, MD: Johns Hopkins University Press, 2004.

Rachels, James. *The End of Life: Euthanasia and Morality.* Oxford: Oxford University Press, 1986.

Rehmann-Sutter, Christoph, et al., eds. *Beihilfe zum Suizid in der Schweiz: Beiträge aus Ethik, Recht und Medizin.* Bern: Peter Lang, 2008.

Rosenfeld, Barry. *Assisted Suicide and the Right to Die: The Interface of Social Science, Public Policy, and Medical Ethics.* Washington, DC: American Psychological Association, 2004.

Rurup, Mette. *Setting the Stage for Death: New Themes in the Euthanasia Debate.* Amsterdam: M.L. Rump, 2005.

Schotmans, Paul, and Tom Meulenbergs. *Euthanasia and Palliative Care in the Low Countries.* Leuven: Peeters, 2005.

Snyder, Lois, and Arthur L. Kaplan. *Assisted Suicide: Finding Common Ground.* Bloomington: Indiana University Press, 2002.

Task Force to Improve the Care of Terminally Ill Oregonians. *The Oregon Death with Dignity Act: A Guidebook for Health Care Providers.* Portland: Oregon Health Sciences University, 1998.

Thomasma, David C. *Asking to Die: Inside the Dutch Debate about Euthanasia.* The Hague: Kluge Academic Publishers, 1998.

Tolmein, Oliver. *Keiner stirbt für sich: Sterbehilfe, Pflegenotstand und das Recht auf Selbstbestimmung.* Munich: C. Bertelsmann, 2006.

Urofsky, Melvin I. *Lethal Judgments: Assisted Suicide and American Law.* Lawrence: University Press of Kansas, 2000.

U.S. Department of Commerce. *Statistical Abstract of the United States: 2004-2005.* Washington, DC: Government Printing Office, 2004.

Wennberg, Robert N. *Terminal Choices: Euthanasia, Suicide and the Right to Die.* Grand Rapids, MI: William B. Eerdmans, 1989.

Articles

Adams, Maurice. "Euthanasia in the Low Countries: Comparative Reflections on the Belgian and Dutch Euthanasia Act." In *Euthanasia and Palliative Care in the Low Countries*, edited by Paul Schotsmans and Tom Meulenbergs (Leuven: Peters, 2005), pp. 5–33.

———. "Euthanasia: The Process of Legal Change in Belgium – Reflections on the Parliamentary Debate." In *Regulating Physician-negotiated Death*, edited by Albert Klijn, et al. ('s-Gravenhage: Elsevier, 2001), pp. 29–47.

Asch, David A. "The Role of Critical Care in Euthanasia and Assisted Death." *New England Journal of Medicine* 334 (1996): 1374–79.

Back, Anthony L. et al. "Physician-assisted Suicide and Euthanasia in Washington State: Patient Requests and Physician Responses." *Journal of the American Medical Association* 275 (1996): 919–25.

Banwink, Marjolein, et al. "Psychiatric Consultation and Quality-of-Life Decision Making in Euthanasia." *The Lancet* 356 (2000): 2067–68.

Baron, Charles. "Hastening Death: The Seven Deadly Sins of the Status Quo." In *Physician-assisted Dying: The Case for Palliative Care and Patient Choice*, edited by Timothy Quill and Margaret Battin (Baltimore, MD: Johns Hopkins University Press, 2004), pp. 309–21.

Battin, Margaret P. "New Life in the Assisted Death Debate in the United States: Scheduled Drugs and NuTech." In *Regulating Physician-*negotiated *Death*, edited by Albert Klijn, et al. ('s-Gravenhage: Elsevier, 2001), pp. 49–63.

Baumann, Peter. "Beihilfe zum Suzid kann eine ärztliche Handlung sein." *Schweizerische Ärztezeitung* 82 (2001): 296–98.

Baumann-Hölzle, Ruth. "Der Tod also Freund: Suizidwunsch einer psychiatrisch erkrankten Patientien." *Schweizerische Ärztezeitung* 84 (2003): 2425–28.

Bernheim, Jan, et al. "Development of Palliative Care and Legalization of Euthanasia: Antagonism or Synergy?" *British Medical Journal* 336 (2008): 864–67.

Bilsen, Johan, et al. "The Incidence and Characteristics of End-of-Life Decisions by GPs in Belgium (Flanders)." *Family Practice* 21 (2004): 282–89.

Blank, Karen, et al. "Instability of Attitudes About Euthanasia and Physician-assisted Suicide in Depressed Older Hospitalized Patients." *General Hospital Psychiatry* 23 (2001): 326–32.

Block, Lieve van den. "End-of-Life Decisions Among Cancer Patients Compared with Noncancer Patients in Flanders, Belgium." *Journal of Clinical Oncology* 24 (2006): 2842–48.

———. "Euthanasia and other End-of Life Decisions: A Mortality Follow-back Study in Belgium." *BMC Public Health* 9 (2009): 79–89.

Block, Susan D., and Andrew Billings. "Patient Requests for Euthanasia in Terminal Illness: The Role of the Psychiatrist." *Psychosomatics* 36 (1995): 445–57.

Boss hard, George, et al. "Foregoing Treatment at the End-of-Life in 6 European Countries." *Archives of Internal Medicine* 165 (2005): 401–07.

———. "A Role for Doctors in Assisted Dying? An Analysis of Legal Regulations and Medical Professional Positions in Six European Countries." *Journal of Medical Ethics* 34 (2008): 28–32.

———. "748 Cases of Suicide Assisted by a Swiss Right-to-Die Organization." *Swiss Medical Weekly* 133 (2003): 310–17.

———. "Sterbeassistenz und die Rolle des Arztes." *Aktuelle Juristische Praxis* 11 (2002): 409–13.

———. "Die Tätigkeit der Sterbehilfeorganisationen und die Rolle des Arztes." In *Beihilfe zum Suizid in der Schweiz: Beiträge aus Ethik, Recht und Medizin,* edited by Christoph Rehmann-Sutter, et al. (Bern: Peter Lang, 2008), pp. 21–30.

Broeckaert, Bert. "Belgium: Toward a Legal Recognition of Euthanasia." *European Journal of Health Law* 8 (2001): 95–107.

Broekaert, Bert, and Rien Janssens. "Palliative Care and Euthanasia: Belgian and Dutch Perspectives." In *Euthanasia and Palliative Care in the Low Countries,* edited by Paul Schotsmans and Tom Meulenbergs (Leuven: Peters, 2005), pp. 35–69.

Buisseret, Caroline, et al. "Palliative Care Associations: The Belgian Experience." *European Journal of Palliative Care* 10 (2003): 247–94.

Burkhardt, Sandra, et al. "Assistance au suicide en Suisse: La position des médecins." *Revue Médicale Suisse* 137 (December 12, 2007): 2861–64.

———. "L'assistance au suicide en Suisse romande: Une etude sur cinq ans." *Journal de Médicine Légale Droit Médical* 50 (2007): 41–44.

Campbell, Eric G., et al. "Professionalism in Medicine: Results of National Survey of Physicians." *Annals of Internal Medicine* 147 (2007): 795–802.

Canetto, Sylvia S., and Janet D. Hollenshead. "Gender and Physician-assisted Suicide: An Analysis of the Krevorkian Cases, 1990-1997." *Omega: The Journal of Death and Dying* 40 (1999-2000): 165–208.

Carlson, Bryant, et al. "Oregon Hospice Chaplains' Experience with Patients Requesting Physician-assisted Suicide." *Journal of Palliative Medicine* 8 (2005): 1160–66.

Chin, Arthur E., et al. "Legalized Physician-assisted Suicide in Oregon: The First Year's Experience." *New England Journal of Medicine* 340 (1999): 577–83.

Cohen, Jonathan. "Influence of Physicians' Life Stances on Attitudes to End-of-Life Decisions and Actual End-of-Life Decisions in Six Countries." *Journal of Medical Ethics* 4 (2008): 247–53.

Cohen-Almagor. "Dutch Perspectives on Palliative Care in the Netherlands." *Issues in Law and Medicine* 18 (2002): 111–26.

Cuperus-Bosma, Jacqueline M. "Assessment of Physician-assisted Death by Members of the Public Prosecution in the Netherlands." *Journal of Medical Ethics* 25 (1999): 8–15.

———. "Physician-assisted Death: Policy-making by the Assembly of Prosecutors-General in the Netherlands." *European Journal of Health Law* 4 (1997): 225–38.

Cuttini, Marina, et al. "End-of-Life Decisions in Neonatal Intensive Care: Physicians' Self-reported Practices in Seven European Countries." *The Lancet* 355 (2000): 2112–18.

Delden, Johannes M. van, et al. "Do-Not-Resuscitate Decisions in Six European Countries." *Critical Care Medicine* 34 (2006): 1686–90.

———. "Slippery Slopes in Flat Countries: A Response." *Journal of Medical Ethics* 25 (1999): 22–24.

———. "The Unfeasibility of Requests for Euthanasia in Advance Directives." *Journal of Medical Ethics* 30 (2004): 447–51.

Deliens, Luc, et al. "Similaritudes et différences entre les loi belge et néélandaire relatives à l'euthanasie." *Revue Médicale de Liège* 58 (2003): 485–92.

———. "End-of-Life Decisions in Medical Practice in Flanders, Belgium: A Nationwide Survey." *The Lancet* 356 (2000): 1806–11.

Dobscha, Steven K. "Oregon Physicians' Responses to Requests for Assisted Suicide: A Qualitative Study." *Journal of Palliative Medicine* 7 (2004): 451–61.

Emanuel, Ezekiel J. "Attitudes and Desires Related to Euthanasia and Physician-assisted Suicide Among Terminally Ill Patients and Their Caregivers." *Journal of the American Medical Association* 284 (2000): 2460–68.

———. "Euthanasia and Physician-assisted Suicide: Attitudes and Experiences of Oncology Patients, Oncologists, and the Public." *The Lancet* 347 (1996): 1805–10.

———. "Euthanasia and Physician-assisted Suicide: A Review of the Empirical Data from the United States." *Archives of Internal Medicine* 162 (2002): 142–52.

Emanuel, Linda L. "A Question of Balance." In *Regulating How We Die: The Ethical, Medical, and Legal Issues Surrounding Physician-assisted Suicide*, edited by Linda L. Emanuel (Cambridge, MA: Harvard University Press, 1998), pp. 234–60.

Englert, Marc. "Deux années d'euthanasie dépénalisée en Belgique: Comparaison avec les Pays-Bas – Premier bilan d'une unite de soins palliatifs (Two Years of Legal Practice of Euthanasia in Belgium: Comparison with the Netherlands – First Evaluation in a Palliative Care Unit)." *Revue Médicale de Bruxelles* (2005): 145–52.

Faber-Landendoen, Kathy, and Jason H.T. Karlawish. "Ought Assisted Suicide Be Only Physician Assisted?" In *Assisted Suicide: Finding Common Ground,* edited by Lois Snyder and Arthur L. Kaplan (Bloomington: Indiana University Press, 2002), pp. 44–54.

Farrenkopf, Tony, and James Bryan. "Psychological Consultation Under the Oregon 1994 Death with Dignity Act: Ethics and Procedures." *Professional Psychology: Research and Practice* 30 (1999): 245–49.

Fischer, Susanne. "Suicide Assisted by Two Right-to-Die Organization." *Journal of Medical Ethics* 34 (2008): 810–14.

———. "Swiss Doctors' Attitudes Towards End-of-Life Decisions and Their Determinants: A Comparison of Their Language Regions." *Swiss Medical Weekly* 135 (2005): 370–76.

Frei, Andreas, et al. "Assisted Suicide as Conducted by a 'Right-to-Die' Society in Switzerland: A Descriptive Analysis of 43 consecutive Cases." *Swiss Medical Weekly* 131 (2001): 375–80.

———. "Beihilfe zum Suizid bei psychisch Kranken." *Nervenarzt* 70 (1999): 1014–18.

Ganzini, Linda, et al. "Attitudes of Oregon Psychiatrists Toward Physician-assisted Suicide." *American Journal of Psychiatry* 153 (1996): 1469–75.

———. "Attitudes of Patients with Amyotrophic Lateral Sclerosis and Their Caregivers Toward Assisted Suicide." *New England Journal of Medicine* 339 (1998): 967–73.

———. "Experiences of Oregon Nurses and Social Workers with Hospice Patients Who Requested Assistance with Suicide." *New England Journal of Medicine* 347 (2002): 582–88.

———. "Oregon Physicians' Attitudes About Their Experiences with End-of-Life Care Since Passage of the Oregon Death with Dignity Act." *Journal of the American Medical Association* 285 (2001): 2363–69.

———. "Oregon Physicians' Perceptions of Patients Who Request Assisted Suicide and Their Families." *Journal of Palliative Medicine* 6 (2003): 381–90.

———. "Physicians' Experiences with the Oregon Death with Dignity Act." *New England Journal of Medicine* 342 (2000): 557–63.

———. "Prevalence of Depression and Anxiety in Patients Requesting Physicians' Aid in Dying: Cross-sectional Survey." *British Medical Journal* 337 (2008): 973–75.

Gastmans, Chris, et al. "Facing Requests for Euthanasia: A Clinical Practice Guideline." *Journal of Medical Ethics* 30 (2004): 212–17.

———. "Pluralism and Ethical Dialogue in Christian Health care Institutions: The View of Caritas Catholica Flanders." *Christian Bioethics* 12 (2006): 265–80.

Geest, Sjaak van der. "Ageism and Euthanasia in the Netherlands: Questions and Conjectures," *Mortality* 8 (2003): 296–304.

Georges, Jean-Jacques. "Physicians' Opinions on Palliative Care and Euthanasia in the Netherlands." *Journal of Palliative Medicine* 9 (2006): 1137–44.

Gevers, Sjef, and Johan Legemaate. "Physician-assisted Suicide in Psychiatry: An Analysis of Case Law and Professional Opinions." In *Asking to Die: Inside the Dutch Debate About Euthanasia,* edited by David C Thomasma (Dortrecht: Kluwe Academic Publishers, 1998), pp. 71–91.

Gordijn, Bert, and Rien Janssens. "Euthanasia and Palliative Care in the Netherlands: An Analysis of the Latest Developments." *Health Care Analysis* 12 (2004): 195–207.

Groenewoud, Johanna H., et al. "Clinical Problems with the Performance of Euthanasia and Physician-assisted Suicide in the Netherlands." *New England Journal of Medicine* 342 (2000): 551–56.

———. "A Nation-wide Study of Decisions to Forego Life-prolonging Treatment in Dutch Medical Practice." *Archives of Internal Medicine* 160 (2000): 357–63.

———. "Physician-assisted Death in Psychiatric Practice in the Netherlands." *New England Journal of Medicine* 336 (1997): 1795–1801.

———. "Psychiatric Consultation with Regards to Requests for Euthanasia or Physician-assisted Suicide." *General Hospital Psychiatry* 26 (2004): 323–30.

Guillod, Olivier, and Alice Schmidt. "*European Journal of Health Law* 12 (2005): 25–38.Have, Henk Ten. "End-of-Life Decision Making in the Netherlands." In *End-of-Life Decision Making: A Cross-*National *Survey,* edited by Robert Blank and Janna C. Merrick (Cambridge, MA: MIT Press, 2005), pp. 147–68.

Haverkate, Ilinka, and Gerrit van der Wal. "Dutch Nursing Home Policies and Guidelines on Physician-assisted Death and Decisions to Forego Treatment." *Public Health* 112 (1998): 419–23.

———. "Policies on Assisted Suicide in Dutch Psychiatric Facilities." *Psychiatric Services* 49 (1998): 98–100.

Haverkate, Ilinka, et al. "The Emotional Impact on Physicians of Hastening the Death of a Patient." *Medical Journal of Australia* 175 (2001): 519–22.

———. "Refused and Granted Requests for Euthanasia and Assisted Suicide in the Netherlands: Interview Study with Structural Questionnaire." *British Medical Journal* 321 (2000): 865–66.

Hedberg, Katrina, and Karel Southwick. "Legalized Physician-assisted Suicide in Oregon, 2001." *New England Journal of Medicine* 346 (2002): 450–52.

Hedberg, Katrina, and Susan W. Tolle. "Physician-assisted Suicide and Changes in Care of Dying: The Oregon Perspective." In *Assisted Suicide: Finding Common Ground,* edited by Lois Snyder and Arthur L. Kaplan (Bloomington: Indiana University Press, 2002), pp. 7–16.

Heide, Agnes van der, et al. "Doctor-assisted Dying: What Difference Does Legalization Make?" *The Lancet* 364 (2004): 24–25.

———. "End-of-Life Practices in the Netherlands Under the Euthanasia Act." *New England Journal of Medicine* 356 (2007): 1957–65.

———. "Medical End-of-Life Decisions in Neonates and Infants in the Netherlands." *The Lancet* 350 (1997): 251–55.

Hendin, Herbert. "The Dutch Experience." *Issues in Law and Medicine* 17 (2002): 223–46.

Hickman, Susan E. "Physicians' and Nurses' Perspectives on Increased Family Reports of Pain in Dying Hospitalized Patients." *Journal of Palliative Medicine* 3 (2000): 413–18.

Hilden, Joanne M. "Attitudes and Practices Among Pediatric Oncologists Regarding End-of-Life Care: Results of the 1998 American Society of Clinical Oncology Survey." *Journal of Clinical Oncology* 19 (2001): 205–12.

Hurst, Samia A., and Alex Mauron. "Assisted Suicide and Euthanasia in Switzerland: Allowing a Role for Non-Physicians." *British Medical Journal* 326 (2003): 271–73.

Huxtable, Richard, and Alastair Campbell. "Palliative Care and the Euthanasia Debate: Recent Developments." *Palliative Medicine* 17 (2003): 94–96.

Huxtable, Richard, and Maaike Möller. "Setting a Principled Boundary? Euthanasia as a Response to 'Life Fatigue.'" *Bioethics* 21 (2007): 117–26.

Jackson, W. Clay. "Palliative Sedation vs. Terminal Sedation: What's in a Name?" *American Journal of Hospice and Palliative Care* 19 (2002): 81–82.

Jans, Jan. "Churches in the Low Countries on Euthanasia: Background, Argumentation and Community." In *Euthanasia and Palliative Care in the Low Countries*, edited by Paul Schotmans and Tom Meulenbergs (Leuven: Peeters, 2005), pp. 175–204.

Jansen van der Weide, Marijke C., et al. "Granted, Undecided, Withdrawn, and Refused Requests for Euthanasia and Physician-assisted Suicide." *Archives of Internal Medicine* 165 (2005): 1698–1704.

———. "Implementation of the Project 'Support and Consultation on Euthanasia in the Netherlands.'" *Health Policy* 69 (2004): 365–73.

———. "Quality of Consultation and the Project 'Support and Consultation in the Netherlands (SCEN).'" *Health Policy* 80 (2007): 97–106.

———. "Requests for Euthanasia and Physician-assisted Suicide and the Availability and Application of Palliative Care Options." *Palliative Supportive Care* 4 (2006): 399–406.

Janssens, Rien J.P.A. "The Concept of Palliative Care in the Netherlands." *Palliative Medicine* 15 (2001): 481–86.

Jannsens, Rien, et al. "Hospice and Euthanasia in the Netherlands: An Ethical Point of View." *Journal of Medical Ethics* 25 (1999): 408–12.

Jochemsen, Henk. "Dutch Court Decisions on Nonvoluntary Euthanasia Critically Reviewed." *Issues in Law and Medicine* 13 (1998): 447–59.

———. "Life-prolonging and Life-terminating Treatment of Severely Handicapped Newborn Babies." *Issues in Law and Medicine* 8 (1992): 167ff. (consulted copy had pagination 1–14).

Kerkhof, A.J.F.M. "How to Deal with Requests for Assisted Suicide: Some Experiences and Practical Guidelines from the Netherlands." *Psychology, Public Policy, and the Law* 6 (2000): 452–66.

Kimsma, Gerritt K., and Evert van Leeuwen. "Euthanasia and Assisted Suicide in the Netherlands and the U.S.A: Comparing Practices, Justifications and Key Concepts in Bioethics and Law." In *Asking to Die: Inside the Dutch Debate about Euthanasia*, edited by David C. Thomasma (Dortrecht: Kluwe Academic Publishers, 1998), pp. 35–70.

———. "Shifts in the Direction of Dutch Bioethics: Forward or Backwards?" *Cambridge Quarterly of Health care Ethics* 14 (2005): 292–97.

Klijn, Albert. "Will Doctors' Behaviour Be More Accountable Under the new Dutch Regime? Reporting and Consultations as Forms of Legal Control." In *Regulating Physician*-Negotiated *Death*, edited by Albert Klijn, et al. ('s-Gravenhage: Elsevier, 2001), pp. 157–78.

Lee, Barbara Coombs, et al. "Physician Assisted Suicide." In *Oregon Health Care Manual*. Vol. 2: *Life and Death Decisions* (Lake Oswego: Oregon State Bar Committee on Continuing Legal Education, 1997), pp. 8-1–8-23.

KNMG (Royal Dutch Medical Association). "Guidelines for Euthanasia." *Issues in Law and Medicine* 3 (1988): 429–37.

Kollée, Louis A.A. "Current Concepts and Future Research on End-of-Life Decision Making in Neonatology in the Netherlands." In *Clinical and Epidemiological Aspects of End-of-Life Decision Making*, edited by Agnes van der Heide, et al. (Amsterdam: Royal Dutch Academy of Arts and Sciences, 2001), pp. 185–96.

Kuin, Annemieke, et al. "Palliative Care Consultation in the Netherlands: A Nationwide Evaluation Study." *Journal of Pain and Symptom Management* 27 (2004): 53–60.

Lau, H.S., et al. "A Nationwide Study on the Practice of Euthanasia and Physician-assisted Suicide in Community and Hospital Pharmacies in the Netherlands." *Pharmacy World and Science* 22 (2000): 3–9.

Lee, Barbara Coombs. "Physician-assisted Suicide." In *Oregon Health Law Manual*. Vol. 2: *Life and Death Decisions*, edited by Theodore C. Falk (Lake Oswego: Oregon State Bar Committee on Continuing Legal Education, 1997), pp. 8-1–8-23.

Lee, Marije L. van der. "Euthanasia and Depression: A Prospective Cohort Study Among Terminally Ill Cancer Patients." *Journal of Clinical Oncology* 23 (2005): 6607–12.

Lee, Melinda A., and Susan W. Tolle. "Oregon's Assisted Suicide Vote: The Silver Lining." *Annals of Internal Medicine* 124 (1996): 267–69.

Legemaate, Johan. "Twenty-five Years of Dutch Experience and Policy on Euthanasia and Assisted Suicide: An Overview." In *Asking to Die: Inside the Dutch Debate about Euthanasia*, edited by David C. Thomasma (Dortrecht: Kluwe Academic Publishers, 1998), pp. 19–34.

Lemiengre, Joke. "Ethics Policies on Euthanasia in Nursing Homes: A Survey in Flanders, Belgium." *Social Science and Medicine* 66 (2008): 376–86.

Lewis, Penney. "The Empirical Slippery Slope from Voluntary to Non-Voluntary Euthanasia." *Journal of Law, Medicine and Ethics* 35 (2007): 197–210.

Löfmark, Rurik, et al. "Palliative Care Training: A Survey Among Physicians in Australia and Europe." *Journal of Palliative Care* 22 (2006): 105–10.

Maas, Paul J. van der. "Changes in Dutch Opinion on Active Euthanasia, 1966 Through 1991." *Journal of the American Medical Association* 273 (1995): 1411–14.

———. "Euthanasia and Other Medical Decisions Concerning the End of Life." *The Lancet* 338 (1991): 669–74.

———. "Euthanasia, Physician-assisted Suicide, and Other Medical Practices Involving the End-of-Life in the Netherlands, 1990-1995." *New England Journal of Medicine* 335 (1996): 1699–1705.

Marcus, Kristine Carlson. "Pharmacists' Response to Oregon's Death with Dignity Act." In *Drug Use in Assisted Suicide and Euthanasia*, edited by Margaret P. Battin and Arthur G. Lipman (New York: Haworth Press, 1996), pp. 151–76.

Matzo, Marianne LaPorte, and Ezchiel J. Emanuel. "Oncology Nurses' Practices of Assisted Suicide and Patient-requested Euthanasia." *Oncology Nurses Forum* 24 (1997): 1725–32.

Meadow, William, and John Lantos. "Epidemiology and Ethics in the NICU." In *Clinical and Epidemiological Aspects of End-of-Life Decision Making*, edited by Agnes van der Heide, et al. (Amsterdam: Royal Dutch Academy of Arts and Sciences, 2001), pp. 177–84.

Meier, Diane E. "A National Survey of Physician-assisted Suicide and Euthanasia in the United States." *New England Journal of Medicine* 338 (1998): 1193–1201.

Miller, Franklin G. "Can Physician-assisted Suicide be Regulated Effectively?" *Journal of Law, Medicine and Ethics* 24 (1996): 225–32.

———. "Regulating Physician-assisted Death." *New England Journal of Medicine* 331 (1994): 119–23.

Miller, Lois L. "Attitudes and Experiences of Oregon Hospice Nurses and Social Workers Regarding Assisted Suicide." *Palliative Medicine* 18 (2004): 685–91.

Nuland, Sherwin B. "Physician-assisted Suicide and Euthanasia in Practice." *New England Journal of Medicine* 342 (2000): 583–84.

Ogden, Russell D. "Non-Physician Assisted Suicide: The Technological Imperative of the Deathing Counterculture." *Death Studies* 25 (2001): 387–401.

Okie, Susan. "Physician-assisted Suicide: Oregon and Beyond." *New England Journal of Medicine* 352 2005): 1627–30.

Onwuteaka-Philipsen, Bregje D. "Dutch Experience of Monitoring Euthanasia." *British Medical Journal* 331 (2005): 691–93.

———. "Euthanasia and Other End-of-Life Decisions in the Netherlands in 1990, 1995 and 2001." *The Lancet* 362 (2003): 395–99.

———. "Euthanatics: Implementation of Protocol to Standardize Euthanasia Among Pharmacists and GPs." *Patient Education and Counseling* 1 (1997): 131–37.

Orentlicher, David. "The Supreme Court and Physician-assisted Suicide: Rejecting Assisted Suicide but Embracing Euthanasia." *New England Journal of Medicine* 337 (1997): 1236–39.

Otlowski, Margaret. "The Effectiveness of Legal Control of Euthanasia: Lessons from Comparative Law." In *Regulating Physician-*negotiated *Death,* edited by Albert Klijn, et al. ('s-Gravenhage: Elsevier, 2001), pp. 137–55.

Passic, Steven D. "Oncologists' Recognition of Depression in Their Patients with Cancer." *Journal of Clinical Oncology* 16 (1998): 1594–1600.

Persels, Jim. "Forcing the Issue of Physician-assisted Suicide: Impact of the Krevorkian Case on the Euthanasia Debate." *Journal of Legal Medicine* 14 (1993): 93–124.

Pereira, J., et al. "The Response of a Swiss Hospital's Palliative Care Consult Team to Assisted Suicide within the Institution." *Palliative Medicine* 22 (2008): 659–67.

Peruzzi, Nico, et al. "Physician-assisted Suicide: The Role of Mental Health Professionals." *Ethics and Behavior* 6 (1996): 353–66.

Pijnenborg, Loes, et al. "Life-terminating Acts Without Explicit Request of Patient." *The Lancet* 341 (1993): 1196–99.

Poenisch, Carol. "Merian Frederick's Story." *New England Journal of Medicine* 339 (1998): 996–98.

Quill, Timothy. "Death and Dignity: A Case of Individualize Decision Making." *New England Journal of Medicine* 324 (1991): 691–94.

———. "The Debate over Physician-assisted Suicide: Empirical Debate and Convergent Views." *Annals of Internal Medicine* 128 (1998): 552–58.

———. "Legal Regulation of Physician-assisted Death: The Latest Report Cards." *New England Journal of Medicine* 356 (2007): 1911–13.

———. "Palliative Treatments of Last Resort: Choosing the Least Harmful Alternative." *Annals of Internal Medicine* 132 (2000): 488–93.

Rietjens, Judith A.C., et al. "A Comparison of Attitudes Towards End-of-Life Decisions: Survey Among the Dutch General Public and Physicians." *Social Science and Medicine* 61 (2005): 1723–32.

———. "Continuous Deep Sedation for Patients Nearing Death in the Netherlands: Descriptive Study." *British Medical Journal* 336 (2008): 810–13.

———. "Terminal Sedation and Euthanasia: A Comparison of Clinical Practice." *Archives of Internal Medicine* 166 (2006): 749–53.

———. "Using Drugs to End Life Without an Explicit Request of the Patient." *Death Studies* 31 (2007): 205–21.

Rietjens, Agnes. "Preferences of the Dutch General Public for a Good Death and Associations with Attitudes Towards End-of-Life Decision-making." *Palliative Medicine* 20 (2006): 685–92.

Rippe, Klaus-Peter, et al. "Urteilsfähigkeit von Menschen mit psychischen Störungen und Suizidbeihilfe." *Schweizerische Juristen-Zeitung* 101 (2005): 53–62, 81–91.

Schmidt, Terri A. "The Physician Orders for Life-sustaining Treatment Program: Oregon Emergency Medical Technicians' Practical Experiences and Attitudes." *Journal of American Geriatrics Society* 52 (2004): 1430–34.

Schoevers, Robert A., et al. "Physician-assisted Suicide in Psychiatry: Developments in the Netherlands." *Psychiatric Services* 49 (1998): 1475–80.

Seymour, Jane E., et al. "Relieving Suffering at the End of Life: Practitioners Perspectives on Palliative Sedation from Three European Countries." *Social Science and Medicine* 64 (2007): 1679–91.

Sheldon, Tony. "'Terminal Sedation' Different from Euthanasia, Dutch Ministers Agree." *British Medical Journal* 327 (2003): 465.

Steen, Jenny van der, et al. "End-of-Life Decision Making in Nursing Home Residents with Dementia and Pneumonia: Dutch Physicians' Intentions Regarding Hastening Death." *Alzheimer Disease and Associated Disorders* 19 (2005): 148–55.

Stell, Lance K. "Physician-assisted Suicide: To Decriminalize or to Legalize, That Is the Question." In *Physician-assisted Suicide: Expanding the Debate*, edited by Margaret Pabst Battin, et al. (New York: Routledge, 1998), pp. 225–51.

Strnad, J., et al. "Suizide in der stationären Psychiatrie unter Beihilfe einer Sterbehilfevereinigung: Fälle aktiver Sterbehilfe?" *Der Nervenarzt* 70 (1999): 645–49.

Sullivan, Amy. D. "Legalized Physician-assisted Suicide in Oregon: The Second Year." *New England Journal of Medicine* 342 (2000): 598–604.

Task Force on Physician-assisted Suicide of the Society for Health and Human Values. "Physician-assisted Suicide: Towards Comprehensive Understanding." *Academic Medicine* 70 (1995): 583–90.

Tibbals, James. "Legal Basis for Ethical Withholding and Withdrawing Life-sustaining Medical Treatment from Infants and Children." *Journal of Pediatrics and Child Health* 43 (2007): 230–36.

Tolle, Susan W., et al. "Characteristics and Proportion of Dying Oregonians Who Personally Consider Physician-assisted Suicide." *Journal of Clinical Ethics* 15 (2004): 111–18.

Tulsky, James A., et al. "Responding to Legal Requests for Physician-assisted Suicide." *Annals of Internal Medicine* 132 (2000): 494–99.

U.S. Department of Justice. "Dispensing of Controlled Substances to Assist Suicide." *Issues in Law and Medicine* 17 (2002): 265–92.

Verhagen, Eduard, and Pieter J.J. Saver. "The Groningen Protocol: Euthanasia in Severely Ill Newborns." *New England Journal of Medicine* 352 (2005): 959–62.

Visser, Jacob J.F., and Herman H. van der Kloot Meisburg. "The Long Road to Legalizing Physician-assisted Death in the Netherlands." *Illness, Crisis, and Law* 11 (2003): 113–21.

Wal, Gerrit van der. "Euthanasia and Assisted Suicide II: Do Dutch Family Doctors Act Prudently?" *Family Practice* 9 (1992): 135–40.

———. "Unrequested Termination of Life: Is It Permissible?" *Bioethics* 7 (1993): 330–39.

Wal, Gerritt van der, and P.J. van der Maas. "Empirical Research on Euthanasia and Other Medical End-of-Life Decisions and the Euthanasia Notification Procedure." In *Asking to Die: Inside the Dutch Debate About Euthanasia,* edited by David C. Thomasma, et al. (Dortrecht: Kluwe Academic Publishers, 1998), pp. 149–83.

Wal, Gerritt van der, et al. "Evaluation of the Notification Procedure for Physician-assisted Death in the Netherlands." *New England Journal of Medicine* 335 (1996): 1706–11.

Widdershoven, Guy A.M. "Beyond Autonomy and Beneficence: The Moral Basis of Euthanasia in the Netherlands." In *Euthanasia and Palliative Care in the Low Countries,* edited by Paul Schotmans and Tom Meulenbergs (Leuven: Peeters, 2005), pp. 83–93.

———. "Euthanasia in the Netherlands: Experience in a Review Committee." *Medicine and Law* 23 (2004): 687–91.

Wineberg, Howard, and James L. Werth, Jr. "Physician-assisted Suicide in Oregon: What Are the Key Factors?" *Death Studies* 27 (2003): 501–18.

Wingfield, Katherine Ann, and Carl S. Hacker. "Physician-assisted Suicide: An Assessment and Comparison of Statutory Approaches Among the States." *Seton Hall Legislative Journal* 32 (2007): 13–64.

Zaré, Maryan, et al. "L'assistance au suicide en Suisse dans la contexte de polypathologie invalidante irréversible." *Revue Médicale Suisse,* no. 128 (October 10, 2007): 2303–2305.

Ziegler, Stephen, and George Bosshard. "Role of Non-governmental Organizations in Physician-assisted Suicide." *British Medical Journal* 334 (2007): 295–98.

Zylicz, Zbigniew. "Palliative Care and Euthanasia in the Netherlands: Observations of a Dutch Physician." In *The Case Against Assisted Suicide: For the Right to End-of-Life Care,* edited by Kathleen Foley and Herbert Hendin. (Baltimore, MD: Johns Hopkins University Press, 2002), pp. 122–43.

INDEX